Department of Veterans Affairs
Health Services Research & Development Service | Evidence-based Synthesis Program

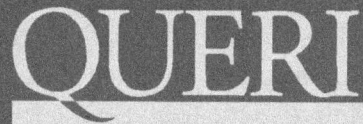

Maintaining Research Integrity: A Systematic Review of the Role of the Institutional Review Board in Managing Conflict of Interest

May 2012

Prepared for:
Department of Veterans Affairs
Veterans Health Administration
Quality Enhancement Research Initiative
Health Services Research & Development Service
Washington, DC 20420

Prepared by:
Evidence-based Synthesis Program (ESP) Center
West Los Angeles VA Medical Center
Los Angeles, CA
Paul G. Shekelle, MD, PhD, Director

Investigators:
Principal Investigator:
Paul G. Shekelle, MD, PhD, Director

Co-Investigators:
Alicia Ruelaz, MD
Isomi M. Miake-Lye, BA

Research Associate:
Jessica M. Beroes, BS

Medical Editor:
Sydney Newberry, PhD

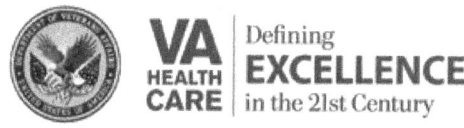

PREFACE

Quality Enhancement Research Initiative's (QUERI) Evidence-based Synthesis Program (ESP) was established to provide timely and accurate syntheses of targeted healthcare topics of particular importance to Veterans Affairs (VA) managers and policymakers, as they work to improve the health and healthcare of Veterans. The ESP disseminates these reports throughout VA.

QUERI provides funding for four ESP Centers and each Center has an active VA affiliation. The ESP Centers generate evidence syntheses on important clinical practice topics, and these reports help:

- develop clinical policies informed by evidence,
- guide the implementation of effective services to improve patient outcomes and to support VA clinical practice guidelines and performance measures, and
- set the direction for future research to address gaps in clinical knowledge.

In 2009, the ESP Coordinating Center was created to expand the capacity of QUERI Central Office and the four ESP sites by developing and maintaining program processes. In addition, the Center established a Steering Committee comprised of QUERI field-based investigators, VA Patient Care Services, Office of Quality and Performance, and Veterans Integrated Service Networks (VISN) Clinical Management Officers. The Steering Committee provides program oversight, guides strategic planning, coordinates dissemination activities, and develops collaborations with VA leadership to identify new ESP topics of importance to Veterans and the VA healthcare system.

Comments on this evidence report are welcome and can be sent to Nicole Floyd, ESP Coordinating Center Program Manager, at nicole.floyd@va.gov.

Recommended citation: Shekelle PG, Ruelaz A, Miake-Lye IM, Beroes JM, Newberry S. Maintaining Research Integrity: A Systematic Review of the Role of the Institutional Review Board in Managing Conflict of Interest, VA-ESP Project #05-226; 2012.

This report is based on research conducted by the Evidence-based Synthesis Program (ESP) Center located at the West Los Angeles VA Medical Center, Los Angeles, CA funded by the Department of Veterans Affairs, Veterans Health Administration, Office of Research and Development, Quality Enhancement Research Initiative. The findings and conclusions in this document are those of the author(s) who are responsible for its contents; the findings and conclusions do not necessarily represent the views of the Department of Veterans Affairs or the United States government. Therefore, no statement in this article should be construed as an official position of the Department of Veterans Affairs. No investigators have any affiliations or financial involvement (e.g., employment, consultancies, honoraria, stock ownership or options, expert testimony, grants or patents received or pending, or royalties) that conflict with material presented in the report.

TABLE OF CONTENTS

EXECUTIVE SUMMARY
    Background 1
    Methods 1
    Data Synthesis 2
    Peer Review 2
    Results 2
    Summary and Discussion 5
    Recommendations for Future Research 6

INTRODUCTION 7
    Current Issues Involving Institutional Review Boards 7
    Conflict of Interest and Institutional Review Boards 8

METHODS
    Topic Development 10
    Search Strategy 10
    Study Selection 11
    Data Abstraction 11
    Data Synthesis 11
    Peer Review 11

RESULTS
    Literature Flow 12
    Key Question #1: What has been published regarding the IRB and each of the following issues:
- Quality improvement initiatives conducted as research studies and therefore requiring IRB approval
- Managing conflict of interest
- Studies requiring approval of multiple IRBs
- Genetic issues
- Payment to research participants or health care professionals 13

    Key Question #2: What is the actual evidence regarding the issue with the largest literature which may inform VA policy? A Detailed Review of Conflict of Interest Studies 21

SUMMARY AND DISCUSSION 29
    Limitations 31
    Recommendations for Future Research 31

REFERENCES 33

TABLES

Table 1. Multisite Institutional Review Board Challenges Articles 13

Table 2. Excerpts from VHA Handbook 1508.05 15

Table 3. When Quality Improvement Initiatives Are Considered Research Articles 17

Table 4. Payment to Patients Articles 19

Table 5. Genetic Studies Articles 19

Table 6. Miscellaneous Articles 20

FIGURE

Figure 1. Literature Flow 12

APPENDIX A. EVIDENCE TABLES 42

APPENDIX B. PEER REVIEW COMMENTS TABLE 45

EXECUTIVE SUMMARY

BACKGROUND

Ethical integrity in the conduct of health care research is essential for maintaining the public trust and support of such activities. Institutional Review Boards (IRBs) play a critical role in maintaining the ethical integrity of research by reviewing research protocols to ensure, among other things, that research participants receive safe and ethical treatment and provide informed consent, and that the potential for a conflict of interest is minimized. The purpose of this review was to catalog the literature on issues pertaining to IRBs, to identify the issue with the greatest number of published studies which might inform VA policy, and to assess the evidence regarding that issue, which were conflict of interest policies and the activities of the IRB.

METHODS

This project was nominated by Ranjana Banerjea, HSR&D & HSR&D Research Best Practices Workgroup (RGP). The goal was to describe the evidence regarding areas of interest in the ethical conduct of research, with a particular focus on the IRB and quality improvement initiatives. Further discussions resulted in the following key questions:

Key Question #1. What has been published regarding the IRB, and each of the following issues:

- Quality improvement initiatives as research
- Conflict of interest
- Studies requiring approval of multiple IRBs
- Genetic issues

Key Question #2. What is the actual evidence regarding the issue with the largest literature which may inform VA policy?

We searched the PubMed databases from 1/01/2000-2/11/2011 for articles related to our key questions. We limited the search to English language articles using search terms related to institutional review boards, informed consent, data use, conflict of interest, ethics, and quality improvement. We also completed related-article searches on four key articles. We also searched the websites of relevant organizations, including the Association of American Medical Colleges (AAMC), Public Responsibility in Medicine and Research (PRIM&R), and the Association for the Accreditation of Human Research Protection Programs, Inc (AAHRPP).

We screened titles and then abstracts, excluding any article not related to the topics listed in Key Question #1. Full articles that met the inclusion criteria were then sorted into the following categories: multi-center IRB; quality improvement as research; conflicts of interest; payments to patients, providers, or study participants (a potential for conflict of interest); genetics research (this category mostly pertained to data repositories and the ethics of using stored genetic material for subsequent studies); miscellaneous articles pertaining to Key Question #1; background articles; and rejected articles.

DATA SYNTHESIS

After performing the search and sorting the articles that met our inclusion criteria, we then selected for detailed review the area for which we identified the greatest number of relevant published studies and for which no VA policies were already in place. Because of the nature of these studies, no quantitative synthesis was possible; therefore our synthesis is descriptive.

PEER REVIEW

A draft version of this report was reviewed by seven technical experts, as well as VA Central Office leadership. Reviewer comments were addressed and our responses were incorporated in the final report.

RESULTS

We reviewed 4,302 titles and abstracts from the electronic search and an additional 490 from related searches for a total of 4,792 references. After applying inclusion/exclusion criteria at the abstract level, we excluded 4,327 references. We retrieved 163 full-text articles and on the basis of further review, we excluded another 47 references. A total of 116 references were included in the current review.

Key Question #1. What has been published regarding the IRB, and each of the following issues:

- Quality improvement initiatives as research
- Conflict of interest
- Studies Requiring Approval of Multiple IRBs
- Genetic issues

We describe here the results of the search we performed. Our goal for this key question was to provide a broad "lay of the land" picture of the available evidence but not a critical synthesis of the evidence.

Multisite Institutional Review Board Challenges

We identified 41 articles that dealt with the challenges of having to submit a research protocol to IRBs at multiple institutions. Most were descriptive studies of how the same application was reviewed by different IRBs. VA has recently implemented a process whereby multi-site VA studies can be reviewed by a single, centralized IRB. Consequently, a detailed review of this issue would not be helpful to VA. The VA Central IRB does not review all protocols that require multiple IRB review. An issue remains that when a protocol is conducted at both the academic affiliate and VA facility, it has to be reviewed by both institutions unless the VA facility has an arrangement to delegate review to the academic affiliate. Further, industry-sponsored studies require multiple IRB reviews and VA prohibits the use of independent (commercial) IRBs.

When Quality Improvement Initiatives Are Considered Research

Quality improvement is an increasingly important activity for health care organizations and also the subject of scholarly activity. Questions have been asked about what quality improvement activities constitute "research" in the context of requiring approval and oversight by an IRB. We identified 31 publications on this issue. However, because VA has recently developed policy on this issue, a detailed review would not be helpful.

Conflict of Interest
We identified 11 publications that dealt with potential conflict of interest (COI) in research, both by investigators and by IRB members. This issue was the one for which we identified the most articles; therefore we selected it for more detailed review (see Key Question #2).

Payment to Patients
We identified nine publications that dealt with the ethical issues surrounding paying patients to participate in research studies or paying heath care professionals to recruit patients into these studies. Four of these articles were descriptive studies about the payments to patients. Across studies, the amount of payment appeared unrelated to the magnitude of the procedures to be performed or the time to participate in the study. Payments to patients ranged widely, from $5 to $2000, with a median of $155. Two studies by the same investigator assessed the potential reasons for payments to participants. The results indicate that investigators consider various factors in deciding whether and how much to pay study participants.

Genetics
We identified eight publications that dealt with potential ethical issues in genetic studies for which an IRB was asked to rule. These issues consisted of consensus recommendations for informed consent and studies describing variation across institutions in genetic policies.

Miscellaneous
Eighteen publications were potentially relevant to the IRB's role in maintaining research integrity but did not fall into one of the existing categories. These studies were a mix of surveys about ethical issues, particularly challenging scenarios that might require special rules (such as practice-based research networks, palliative care, and nursing research) and methods to evaluate the workings of the IRB.

Key Question #2. Detailed review of Conflict of Interest studies
COI, both financial and non-financial, is increasingly recognized as an important aspect of maintaining public trust in medical research. In reviewing the literature available on COI, we start with those studies that examined the goals of disclosure, in general, as well as what disclosure should include.

Purposes of Disclosure to the IRB
We identified four studies that dealt with the purposes of disclosure. Commonly reported goals included promoting informed decision making, respecting patients' perceived right to know, establishing or maintaining trust, minimizing risk of legal liability, deterring troubling financial relationships, and protecting research participants' welfare.

Who Has Policies around Disclosure?
Three studies were descriptive assessments of various institutions' COI policies. A conclusion common to all three studies was the wide variability in policies among institutions.

Two studies were descriptive assessments of COI policies within a single IRB. Again a common conclusion was variability in the policies.

Persons or Interests Requiring Disclosure

Four studies were descriptive assessments of policies specifying which persons or entities were required to disclose COI. All policies required research investigators to disclose, but beyond that commonality, policies varied substantially on the requirement for family members (i.e., parents, siblings, "de facto spouses," or other family members) of researchers to disclose COI.

Party to Which Disclosure Must Be Made

Five studies reported descriptive assessments of policies regarding the entities to whom disclosure needed to be made. All studies reported that all policies required disclosure to a university or institutional official or committee. Studies disagreed regarding disclosure to the IRB, varying from one percent of institutions requiring "initial" disclosure to the IRB, to 60 percent of the "top 10" National Institutes of Health (NIH)-funded research institutions requiring disclosure to the IRB, to the IRB having "a role" in review of investigators' financial relationships in about 75 percent of institutions. Differences in wording probably account for some of the differences in responses.

One study surveyed IRB chairs about the persons to whom IRB members' COI should be reported. Sixty-two percent answered that their IRB members reported their industry relationships to the IRB chair, 76 percent of respondents reported to the entire IRB, 53 percent of respondents reported to a group or individual within the organization but separate from the IRB, 7 percent reported to an entity external to the IRB and the institution that it serves, and 2 percent reported to an unnamed 'other.'

Managing Disclosure of Potential Conflicts of Interest

One study reported a descriptive assessment of how COI was managed. Within the policies of the 235 medical schools and other research institutions, disclosure was managed by divestment of interest (62 percent), withdrawal of the investigator from the project (61 percent), disclosure to the IRB or research subjects (0 percent), disclosure to the funding agency or sponsor (43 percent), disclosure to journals publishing findings (2 percent), disclosure to collaborating researchers (1 percent), a modification of research plan (59 percent), monitoring of the project (66 percent), requirement for additional peer review (7 percent), or public disclosure (59 percent).

Monitoring Compliance

No studies were identified that described how compliance was monitored.

Managing Noncompliance

Two studies described assessments of policies for managing noncompliance. As with other policies, policies for managing noncompliance varied widely.

Potential Harms of Disclosure

One study surveyed investigators, IRB chairs, and COI Committees about the potential negative effects of disclosure. These effects included the belief that disclosure might affect participant recruitment and enrollment, expressed by 63 percent (5/8) of investigators, 78 percent (18/23) of IRB chairs, and 79 percent (11/14) of COIC chairs; the belief that disclosure 'breaks down trust,' expressed by, respectively, 63 percent, 26 percent, and 21 percent; the belief that disclosure lengthens informed consent documents by, respectively, 38 percent, 26 percent, 29 percent; and the belief that disclosure lengthens the informed consent process, by, respectively, 38 percent, 9 percent, and 0 percent.

SUMMARY AND DISCUSSION

Key Question #1

The topic areas for which the largest number of studies has been published are the challenges of getting multiple IRB approvals for multi-site research studies and defining when quality improvement initiatives are considered research. Both are topic areas for which VA has recently implemented national policies designed to reduce complexity and uncertainty for researchers while maintaining appropriate safeguards for patients. These two topics account for 60 percent of the articles we identified.

Of the remaining studies, the next most common topic of study was COI, which we designated as the focus of key question #2 for an in-depth review. A modest body of research has been devoted to studies of payments to providers or patients for participating in research; these studies indicate wide variability and little relationship between the time expected for participant involvement and the payment.

We also identified a modest number of published studies about the ethics of genetic studies. This finding may be surprising, given the degree of interest in the topic in both professional and lay audiences.

Key Question #2

With regard to COI, we identified a modest number of published studies, almost all of them descriptive and some with substantial limitations (such as low survey response rates or restriction of the sample to a small number of sites). Many more studies have examined COI among research investigators than among IRB members reviewing proposed research. Nevertheless, the available evidence indicates potentially worrisome variation in practice across sites. We identified variation in four domains:

1. Who needs to disclose?
   Which members of the research project need to provide COI disclosures? This group could include principal investigator(s), co-investigators, research assistants, and other research staff.
2. What needs to be disclosed?
   This information includes not only direct financial interests, but also indirect financial support such as support for travel to attend meetings, and non-financial COI.
3. How distant a relationship may an individual have with an investigator and still be

required to disclose COI? This group almost always includes a spouse, but could also include children, parents, siblings, or other extended family members.
4. To whom does the information need to be disclosed? The target could be a specific official or committee of the IRB, or potentially the research participants.

RECOMMENDATIONS FOR FUTURE RESEARCH

Maintaining high ethical standards of conduct in research, both for the investigator and for IRBs, is a high prority for VA, and not one where VA can or should merely react to problems when they are identified. Rather, VA should aim that research conducted at all VA insitutions is held to the same high standard, much as it has done with clinical care over the past 15 years. To do so, VA should:

1. Conduct a descriptive study of current COI practices for investigators and IRB members at all VA facilities,
2. Use this information to determine which areas of current practices have unjustifiable levels of variation across sites,
3. Convene stakeholders to determine best practices for these processes,
4. Create VA-wide policy about these practices, and
5. Monitor implementation across facilities.

As an example, right now it is unknown whether VA facilities vary across the four dimensions of "who should disclose," "what to disclose," "how distant must an individual be related to an investigator to avoid disclosure," and "to whom should COI be disclosed." VA facilities may vary, possibly greatly, in these dimensions. VA has striven to provide, and patients have come to expect, one high standard of clinical care no matter which VA facility they visit. It is unreasonable for Veterans to expect differing ethical standards of research across VA facilities. Research-informed policy can ensure that COI disclosure be made as standard as clinical care, while allowing local flexibility when it is justified. Implicit in this statement is that defining standard COI policies, while a necessary condition, is not sufficient. Monitoring implementation is critical. AAHRPP has attempted to institute a common standard across VA facilities (at least those that are accredited) with response to a single disclosure threshold, disclosure from all individuals involved in the research, and management plans. One challenge is as a government agency VA must follow the government-wide ethics regulations that state federal employees may not have financial interests that relate to their work. All VA IRBs, that are accredited, have conflict of interest policies.

After this uniformity is accomplished, the next step will be to try and provide national VA guidelines on managing COI for individuals (investigators) and IRBs. While preservation of local autonomy is important for providing insitutions with the flexibility they need, some system-wide principles would be useful to help local sites inform COI management decisions. Non-financial COI will also need to be addressed at some point. Given the current imprecision with which non-financial conflicts are defined, the VA would best defer this topic until a greater degree of consensus is reached in the scientific community on how non-financial conflicts are defined.

Lastly, since many VA insitutions that conduct research have university affiliates, a potential complicating factor is the lack of harmony between VA COI and that of these university affliates.

EVIDENCE REPORT

INTRODUCTION

Ethical integrity in the conduct of health care research is essential for maintaining the public trust and support of such activities. Without research, health care cannot advance in a scientific fashion. But by definition, research that involves human participants necessitates that some aspects of their care are no longer being provided solely for their health benefit: research is meant to inform the care of future patients. Therefore, care provided as part of a research protocol always involves a risk of harm. Sometimes it is a direct health risk, as in the case of a new treatment of hoped-for-but-as-yet-unproven benefit with the potential for certain adverse events; or it may be less obvious, such as the risk of disclosure of sensitive information. The ethical management of risk is a primary focus of maintaining integrity in research.

Landmarks in the evolution of ethics for the conduct of research on humans include the 1946 Nuremberg code in response to atrocities committed by Nazi physicians on prisoners, which stated the basic requirement for any such research be "the voluntary consent" of the subjects involved;[1] the Declaration of Helsinki (1964, with subsequent updates) that declared (among other things) that informed consent is necessary, that risks should not exceed benefits, and that research protocols should be reviewed by an independent committee;[2] the exposé by Henry Beecher (1966) of about two dozen "unethical or questionable ethical studies;"[3] and the Belmont Report (1979), which was undertaken in part as the result of the infamous Tuskegee Syphilis study, where curative treatment was withheld from low-income African American males with syphilis.[4] The Belmont Report established the three basic principles of ethical research: respect for persons, beneficence, and justice; and their application to informed consent, assessment of risk and benefits, and the selection of subjects (participants).

In 1966, partly in response to the exposé by Beecher, the United States Public Health Service released a policy statement on ethical conduct of research:

"No new, renewal, or continuation research or research training grant in support of clinical research and investigation involving human beings shall be awarded by the Public Health Service unless the grantee has indicated in the application the manner in which the grantee institution will provide prior review of the judgment of the principal investigator or program director by a committee of his institutional associates."[5]

And thus the Institutional Review Board (IRB) became a requirement for federally funded research.

CURRENT ISSUES INVOLVING INSTITUTIONAL REVIEW BOARDS

In today's research environment, the IRB serves a number of functions, first and foremost being the protection of research participants. This protection includes insurance that potential participants are sufficiently briefed about the nature of the research and their participation that they are able to provide informed consent. The IRB also evaluates the appropriateness of payment for research participation and recruitment. IRBs set policies on the kinds of data that can be collected from participants, e.g., genetic profiles, and how those data must be protected. IRBs also distinguish what activities constitute a research study with human participation from quality improvement initiatives that do not directly involve participants. Researchers as well as IRBs grapple with how to ensure that research conducted at multiple sites or by investigators from multiple institutions adequately protects participants (which often requires review by an IRB at each site or institution). Finally, IRBs assess whether disclosure of potential financial conflicts of interest among research team members is required as part of the management plan when a conflict exists.

CONFLICT OF INTEREST AND INSTITUTIONAL REVIEW BOARDS

The fact that money and reputations depend on the results of some research creates the potential for conflicts of interest (COI). Research investigators who have a financial or non-financial interest in the results of their research may consciously or unconsciously bias the conduct and interpretation of a study to yield their preferred outcome. The issue of COI in medical research has been the subject of countless lay media stories and numerous reports and commissions. One of the most prominent recent reports was from the Institute of Medicine: "Conflict of Interest in Medical Research, Education and Practice." Two of the principle recommendations of the IOM report were as follows:

1. "Institutions that carry out medical research, medical education, clinical care, or practice guideline development should adopt, implement, and make public conflict of interest policies for individuals that are consistent with the other recommendations in this report. To manage identified conflicts of interest and monitor the implementation of management recommendations, institutions should create a conflict of interest committee. That committee should use a full range of management tools, as appropriate, including elimination of the conflicting financial interest, prohibition or restriction of involvement of the individual with a conflict of interest in the activity related to the conflict, and providing additional disclosures of the conflict of interest." (p.18)

2. "The National Institutes of Health should develop rules governing institutional conflicts of interest for research institutions covered by current U.S. Public Health Service regulations. The rules should require the reporting of identified institutional conflicts of interest and the steps that have been taken to eliminate or manage such conflicts."[6] (p. 22)

The considerable potential for COI has been documented numerous times. In a systematic review by Bekelman and colleagues, 37 studies were identified that assessed the extent or impact of financial relationships between industry investigators, and academic institutions.[7] Findings showed that 23 percent to 28 percent of academic investigators received research funding from industry and that many academic institutions had equity positions in start-up companies that sponsor research. Furthermore, industry sponsorship was significantly associated with conclusions favorable to the industry. Similar and more recent results were listed in the IOM report: For example, 27 percent of academic department chairs are paid consultants to industry.[8] The report listed a number of particularly troubling examples of biased reporting in industry-supported clinical research. Also, studies have documented marked variability in the institutional policies regarding COI. In a 1998 survey of 100 leading research institutions in the United States, about half required disclosure by all faculty while another half required disclosure only from principle investigators or those conducting research.[9] This analysis concluded that most policies on COI lack specificity about the kinds of relationships with industry that are permitted or prohibited. Studies have shown variability in how conflict of interest policies are implemented, even within a single university system.[10,11]

The aim of this report was to catalog the literature on issues pertaining to IRBs and the ethical conduct of research, to identify the issue with the greatest number of published studies for which no current VA policy exists, and to assess the evidence regarding that issue, which was policies for minimizing conflict of interest and the activities of the IRB in that regard.

METHODS

TOPIC DEVELOPMENT

This project was nominated by Ranjana Banerjea, HSR&D & HSR&D Research Best Practices Workgroup (RGP). The goal was to describe the evidence regarding areas of interest in the ethical conduct of research, with a particular focus on research and quality improvement initiatives. Further discussions resulted in the following key questions:

Key Question #1. What has been published regarding the IRB and each of the following issues:

- Quality improvement initiatives conducted as research studies and therefore requiring IRB approval
- Managing conflict of interest
- Studies requiring approval of multiple IRBs
- Genetic issues

Key Question #2. What is the actual evidence regarding the issue with the largest literature which may inform VA policy?

SEARCH STRATEGY

Search Terms and Algorithms

"institutional review board" Or "institutional review boards" OR advisory committees OR ethics committee OR ethics committees OR "national commission for the protection of human subjects"
AND
"informed consent"[ti] OR informed consent[mh] OR selection bias OR selection biases OR privacy OR confidentiality OR "using data" OR "data use" OR "data usage" OR "human experimentation" OR "patient safety" OR registry OR registries OR medical records OR ethics[ti] OR ethics[mh] OR ethical* OR "conflict of interest"
AND
qi OR "quality improvement" OR "quality-improvement" OR mortality OR quality assurance, health care OR total quality management OR "quality management" OR quality of health care OR "health care quality" OR quality control
OR quality[ti]

Databases Searched

We searched PubMed databases from 1/01/2000-2/11/2011 for English-language articles related to our key questions. Search terms were chosen that pertained to institutional review boards and informed consent, data use, conflict of interest, ethics, and quality improvement initiatives.

Related Articles Search

We also completed related article searches in Pub Med on four key articles.[12-15]

Internet Search

We searched the websites of relevant organizations, including Association of American Medical Colleges (AAMC), Public Responsibility in Medicine and Research (PRIM&R), the Association for the Accreditation of Human Research Protection Programs, Inc (AAHRPP), and the National Institutes of Health (NIH), for empiric studies of COI.

STUDY SELECTION

We completed a title screen, excluding any article that, from its title alone, indicated it was unrelated to Key Question #1. We then performed another round of screening on the abstracts of articles that passed the first round, again excluding articles not related to Key Question #1. Full articles included from this stage were then categorized according to their topic of interest: the challenges of IRB approval in multi-site studies; when quality improvement initiatives become research; conflicts of interest; payments to patients, providers, or study participants (which we split off from conflicts of interest as it seemed to be a distinctive topic in and of itself); genetics research (this category mainly pertained to data repositories); miscellaneous articles pertaining to Key Question #1; background articles; and articles rejected at that stage as not being relevant. Articles were rejected if the scope was not relevant to our population (e.g. articles about children) or setting (e.g. if the article was not pertinent to IRBs), or if they were commentaries, opinions, or did not present original data, i.e. documents presenting an organizational COI policy or a position paper were rejected.

DATA ABSTRACTION

We coded each article according to the issue it addressed (per Key Question #1) or as "miscellaneous." To the four issues addressed in Key Question #1, we added a 5th category, "payments to patients or providers." For articles about conflict of interest, the topic selected for detailed review, we abstracted information about the study design, participants, and findings, and constructed an evidence table (Appendix A).

DATA SYNTHESIS

After assessing the output of our literature searches, we then selected for detailed review the area that had the greatest number of relevant published studies that did not already have VA policies in place, namely conflict of interest. Because of the nature of these studies, no quantitative synthesis was possible; therefore our synthesis is narrative.

PEER REVIEW

A draft version of this report was reviewed by seven technical experts as well as VA Central Office leadership. Their comments and our responses are presented in Appendix B.

RESULTS

LITERATURE FLOW

We reviewed 4,302 titles and abstracts from the electronic search and an additional 490 from related searches, for a total of 4,792 references. After applying inclusion/exclusion criteria at the title and abstract levels, we excluded 4,327 references. We retrieved 163 full-text articles for further review and excluded another 47 references. We then categorized the remaining 116 included studies by the issue addressed. Issues were not mutually exclusive, and two articles overlapped between the genetics and COI groups. Figure 1 details the exclusion criteria and the number of references related to each of the topics.

Figure 1. Literature Flow

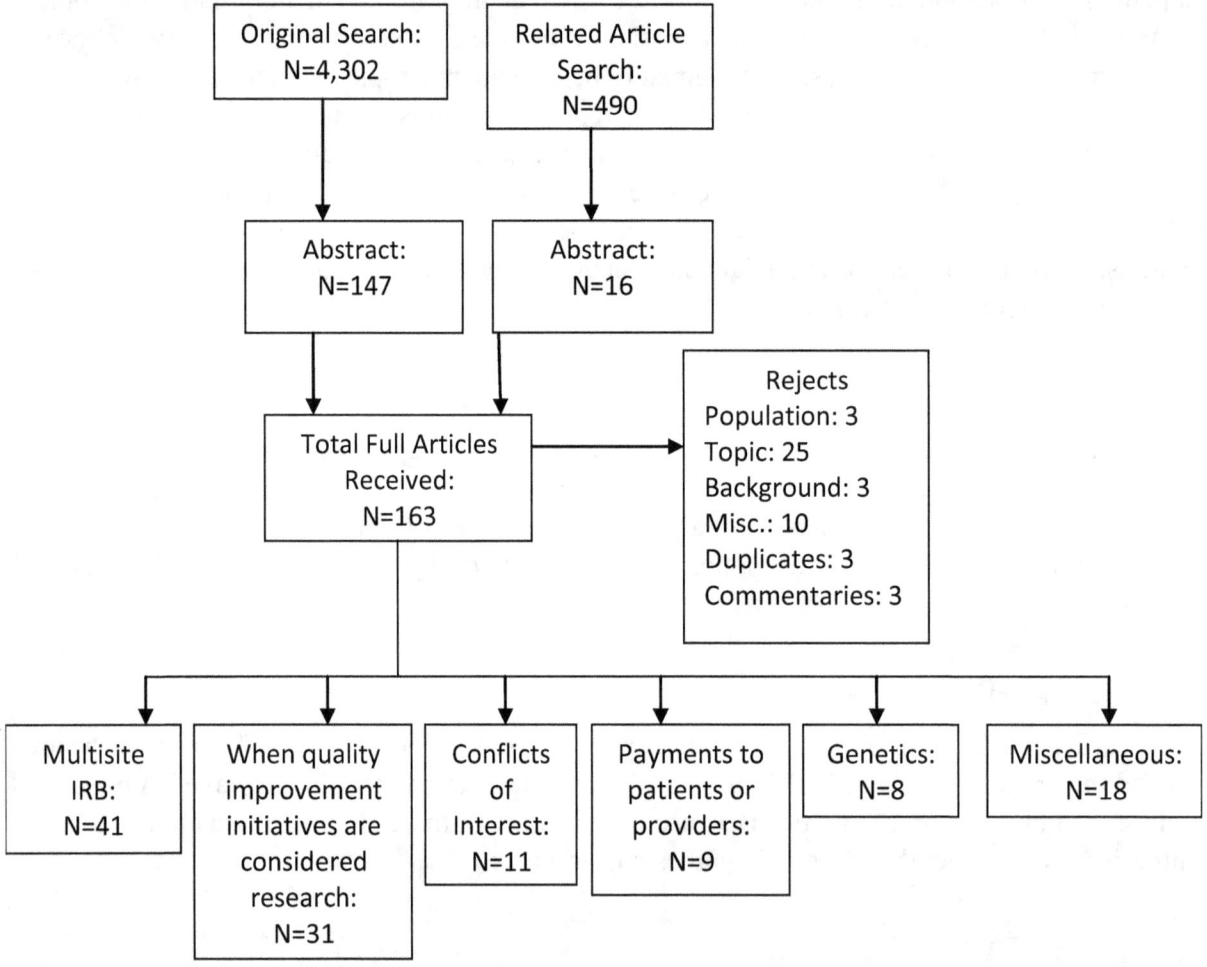

KEY QUESTION #1: What has been published regarding the IRB and each of the following issues:

- Quality improvement initiatives conducted as research studies and therefore requiring IRB approval
- Managing conflict of interest
- Studies requiring approval of multiple IRBs
- Genetic issues
- Payment to research participants or health care professionals

We describe here the results of the brief review we performed. Our goal was to assess the state of the literature on issues pertaining to IRBs and to identify the issue with the largest body of research for which no current VA policy exists.

MULTISITE INSTITUTIONAL REVIEW BOARD CHALLENGES

We identified 41 articles that dealt with the challenges of having to submit a research protocol to IRBs (Table 1) at multiple institutions.[16-56] Most of these were descriptive studies of how the same application was reviewed by different IRBs. In general these studies reported a great deal of variability in the ways the same protocol was reviewed by IRBs at different institutions, and the resources and time lost by investigators dealing with these multiple, and occasionally conflicting requests from different IRBs. VA has recently implemented a process whereby multisite VA studies can be reviewed by a single, centralized IRB. Consequently, this topic was not an area where a detailed review would be most helpful to VA.

Table 1. Multisite Institutional Review Board Challenges Articles

Multisite Institutional Review Board Challenges
Angell E, Sutton AJ, Windridge K, Dixon-Woods M. Consistency in decision making by research ethics committees: a controlled comparison. J Med Ethics 2006;32:662-4.[16]
Blustein J, Regenstein M, Siegel B, Billings J. Notes from the field: jumpstarting the IRB approval process in multicenter studies. Health Serv Res 2007;42:1773-82.[17]
Burman W, Breese P, Weis S, Bock N, Bernardo J, Vernon A. The effects of local review on informed consent documents from a multicenter clinical trials consortium. Control Clin Trials 2003;24:245-55.[18]
Burman WJ, Reves RR, Cohn DL, Schooley RT. Breaking the camel's back: multicenter clinical trials and local institutional review boards. Ann Intern Med 2001;134:152-7.[19]
Christie DR, Gabriel GS, Dear K. Adverse effects of a multicentre system for ethics approval on the progress of a prospective multicentre trial of cancer treatment: how many patients die waiting? Intern Med J 2007;37:680-6.[20]
Dilts DM, Sandler AB. Invisible barriers to clinical trials: the impact of structural, infrastructural, and procedural barriers to opening oncology clinical trials. J Clin Oncol 2006;24:4545-52.[21]
Dyrbye LN, Thomas MR, Mechaber AJ, Eacker A, Harper W, Massie FS, Jr., Power DV, Shanafelt TD. Medical education research and IRB review: an analysis and comparison of the IRB review process at six institutions. Acad Med 2007;82:654-60.[22]
Dziak K, Anderson R, Sevick MA, Weisman CS, Levine DW, Scholle SH. Variations among Institutional Review Board reviews in a multisite health services research study. Health Serv Res 2005;40:279-90.[23]
Edwards SJ, Stone T, Swift T. Differences between research ethics committees. Int J Technol Assess Health Care 2007;23:17-23.[24]
Elwyn G, Seagrove A, Thorne K, Cheung WY. Ethics and research governance in a multicentre study: add 150 days to your study protocol. BMJ 2005;330:847.[25]
Enzle ME, Schmaltz R. Ethics review of multi-centre clinical trials in Canada. Health Law Rev 2005;13:51-7.[26]

Ezzat H, Ross S, von Dadelszen P, Morris T, Liston R, Magee LA. Ethics review as a component of institutional approval for a multicentre continuous quality improvement project: the investigator's perspective. BMC Health Serv Res 2010;10:223.[27]

Gold JL, Dewa CS. Institutional review boards and multisite studies in health services research: is there a better way? Health Serv Res 2005;40:291-307.[28]

Green LA, Lowery JC, Kowalski CP, Wyszewianski L. Impact of institutional review board practice variation on observational health services research. Health Serv Res 2006;41:214-30.[29]

Greene SM, Geiger AM. A review finds that multicenter studies face substantial challenges but strategies exist to achieve Institutional Review Board approval. J Clin Epidemiol 2006;59:784-90.[30]

Greene SM, Geiger AM, Harris EL, Altschuler A, Nekhlyudov L, Barton MB, Rolnick SJ, Elmore JG, Fletcher S. Impact of IRB requirements on a multicenter survey of prophylactic mastectomy outcomes. Ann Epidemiol 2006;16:275-8.[31]

Helfand BT, Mongiu AK, Roehrborn CG, Donnell RF, Bruskewitz R, Kaplan SA, Kusek JW, Coombs L, McVary KT. Variation in institutional review board responses to a standard protocol for a multicenter randomized, controlled surgical trial. J Urol 2009;181:2674-9.[32]

Hicks SC, James RE, Wong N, Tebbutt NC, Wilson K. A case study evaluation of ethics review systems for multicentre clinical trials. Med J Aust 2009;191:280-2.[33]

Koski G, Aungst J, Kupersmith J, Getz K, Rimoin D. Cooperative research ethics review boards: a win-win solution? IRB 2005;27:1-7.[34]

McWilliams R, Hoover-Fong J, Hamosh A, Beck S, Beaty T, Cutting G. Problematic variation in local institutional review of a multicenter genetic epidemiology study. JAMA 2003;290:360-6.[35]

Menikoff J. The paradoxical problem with multiple-IRB review. N Engl J Med 2010;363:1591-3.[36]

Newgard CD, Hui SH, Stamps-White P, Lewis RJ. Institutional variability in a minimal risk, population-based study: recognizing policy barriers to health services research. Health Serv Res 2005;40:1247-58.[37]

Olver IN. A case study evaluation of ethics review systems for multicentre clinical trials. Med J Aust 2010;192:293.[38]

Pogorzelska M, Stone PW, Cohn EG, Larson E. Changes in the institutional review board submission process for multicenter research over 6 years. Nurs Outlook 2010;58:181-7.[39]

Racine E, Bell E, Deslauriers C. Canadian research ethics boards and multisite research: experiences from two minimal-risk studies. IRB 2010;32:12-8.[40]

Ravina B, Deuel L, Siderowf A, Dorsey ER. Local institutional review board (IRB) review of a multicenter trial: local costs without local context. Ann Neurol 2010;67:258-60.[41]

Rikkert MG, Lauque S, Frolich L, Vellas B, Dekkers W. The practice of obtaining approval from medical research ethics committees: a comparison within 12 European countries for a descriptive study on acetylcholinesterase inhibitors in Alzheimer's dementia. Eur J Neurol 2005;12:212-7.[42]

Rose CD. Local vs central institutional review boards for multicenter studies. JAMA 2003;290:2126; author reply 2126-7.[43]

Saginur R, Dent SF, Schwartz L, Heslegrave R, Stacey S, Manzo J. Ontario Cancer Research Ethics Board: lessons learned from developing a multicenter regional institutional review board. J Clin Oncol 2008;26:1479-82.[44]

Sarson-Lawrence M, Alt C, Mok MT, Dodds M, Rosenthal MA. Trust and confidence: towards mutual acceptance of ethics committee approval of multicentre studies. Intern Med J 2004;34:598-603.[45]

Shelby-James T, Agar MR, Currow DC. A case study evaluation of ethics review systems for multicentre clinical trials. Med J Aust 2010;192:292.[46]

Sherwood ML, Buchinsky FJ, Quigley MR, Donfack J, Choi SS, Conley SF, Derkay CS, Myer CM, 3rd, Ehrlich GD, Post JC. Unique challenges of obtaining regulatory approval for a multicenter protocol to study the genetics of RRP and suggested remedies. Otolaryngol Head Neck Surg 2006;135:189-96.[47]

Silverman H, Hull SC, Sugarman J. Variability among institutional review boards' decisions within the context of a multicenter trial. Crit Care Med 2001;29:235-41.[48]

Stair TO, Reed CR, Radeos MS, Koski G, Camargo CA. Variation in institutional review board responses to a standard protocol for a multicenter clinical trial. Acad Emerg Med 2001;8:636-41.[49]

Stark AR, Tyson JE, Hibberd PL. Variation among institutional review boards in evaluating the design of a multicenter randomized trial. J Perinatol 2010;30:163-9.[50]

Tully J, Ninis N, Booy R, Viner R. The new system of review by multicentre research ethics committees: prospective study. BMJ 2000;320:1179-82.[51]

Vick CC, Finan KR, Kiefe C, Neumayer L, Hawn MT. Variation in Institutional Review processes for a multisite observational study. Am J Surg 2005;190:805-9.[52]

Wagner TH, Bhandari A, Chadwick GL, Nelson DK. The cost of operating institutional review boards (IRBs). Acad Med 2003;78:638-44.[53]

Wagner TH, Cruz AM, Chadwick GL. Economies of scale in institutional review boards. Med Care 2004;42:817-23.[54]

Wagner TH, Murray C, Goldberg J, Adler JM, Abrams J. Costs and benefits of the national cancer institute central institutional review board. J Clin Oncol 2010;28:662-6.[55]

Yawn BP, Graham DG, Bertram SL, Kurland MJ, Dietrich AJ, Wollan PC, Brandt EC, Huff JM, Pace WD. Practice-based research network studies and institutional review boards: two new issues. J Am Board Fam Med 2009;22:453-60.[56]

When Quality Improvement Initiatives Are Considered Research

Quality improvement is an increasingly important activity for health care organizations and also the subject of scholarly activity. Questions have been asked about what quality improvement activities constitute "research" and would therefore require approval and oversight by an IRB.[57,60] This issue was highlighted by the controversy over the Keystone Intensive Care Unit project, where a quality improvement project to decrease bloodstream infections was considered by the Johns Hopkins IRB as "exempt" and later over-ruled by the Office for Human Research Protection, which subsequently amended their ruling.[61]

More recently, VA has developed its own definition of what constitutes "research" for this purpose (Table 2).

Table 2. Excerpts from VHA Handbook 1508.05

Generalizable Knowledge: Information that is designed to expand the knowledge base of a scientific discipline (or other scholarly field of study).
Operations Activities: Operations activities are certain administrative, financial, legal, quality assurance, quality improvement, and public health endeavors that are necessary to support VHA's missions of delivering health care to the nation's Veterans, conducting research and development, performing medical education, and contributing to national emergency response. VHA operations activities include (but are not limited to):   (1) Conducting quality assessment and improvement activities; systems redesign activities; population-based activities relating to improving health, ensuring safety, or reducing health care costs; and case management and care coordination.   (2) Reviewing the competence or qualifications of health care professionals; evaluating provider and health plan performance; training health care and non-health care professionals; and accreditation, certification, licensing, or credentialing activities.   (3) Underwriting and other activities relating to the creation, renewal, or replacement of a contract of health insurance or health benefits and ceding, securing, or placing a contract for reinsurance of risk relating to health care claims.   (4) Conducting or arranging for medical review, legal analyses, or auditing services, including fraud and abuse detection and compliance programs.   (5) Business planning and development, such as conducting cost-management and planning analyses related to managing and operating an entity.   (6) Business management and general administrative activities.
Research: Research is a systematic investigation (including research development, testing, and evaluation) <u>designed</u> to develop or contribute to generalizable knowledge by <u>expanding the knowledge base of a scientific discipline</u> (or other scholarly field of study). *NOTE: Research typically involves the testing of concepts by the scientific method of formulating a hypothesis or research question, systematically collecting and recording relevant data, and interpreting the results in terms of the hypothesis or question to <u>expand the knowledge base of a field of study</u>. Research is further discussed in the Federal Policy (Common Rule) for the Protection of Human Subjects at 38 CFR Part 16; in VHA Directive 1200; and in VHA Handbooks 1200.01 and 1200.05.*

> **Systematic Investigation:**
> A systematic investigation is an activity that is planned in advance and that uses data collection and analysis to answer a question. Although research must include systematic investigation, many <u>non-research</u> activities also include systematic investigation. Systematic investigation does not, in and of itself, define research. Examples of systematic investigations, which <u>may or may not</u> constitute research, include (but are not limited to) activities involving:
> 1. Questionnaires or surveys
> 2. Observations
> 3. Focus groups
> 4. Interviews
> 5. Analyses of existing data
> 6. Analyses of biological specimens
> 7. Medical chart reviews
> 8. Epidemiologic reviews or analyses
> 9. Program evaluations
> 10. Quality assessment, quality improvement, and quality management
> 11. Interventional studies
> 12. Clinical trials

These points can also be summed up thus (text courtesy of Mi-Fu Tsan):

Health care operations activities such as quality assurance and quality improvement projects differ from research in that health care operations activities are specifically designed to support the operations of a health care institution, while research is specifically designed to contribute to generalizable knowledge (i.e., to expand the knowledge base of a scientific discipline or other scholarly field of study). Both health care operations activity and research utilize systematic investigation to achieve their objectives. Similar to research, the results of health care operations activity may be published in scientific journals and ultimately expand scientific knowledge base. Thus, neither systematic investigation nor publication effectively distinguishes health care operations activity from research. However, when a health care operations activity goes beyond its purpose of supporting the operations of a health care institution by adding elements specifically designed to expand the knowledge base of a scientific discipline or other scholarly field of study, the activity constitutes research.

We identified 31 publications on this issue (see Table 3).[14, 57-60, 62-87] As VA has already developed policy in this area, this question was not an area for which a detailed review would be helpful.

Table 3. When Quality Improvement Initiatives Are Considered Research Articles

When Quality Improvement Initiatives Are Considered Research
Taylor, H. A., P. J. Pronovost, et al. (2010). "The ethical review of health care quality improvement initiatives: findings from the field." Issue Brief (Commonw Fund) 95: 1-12.[14]
Platteborze, L. S., S. Young-McCaughan, et al. (2010). "Performance Improvement/Research Advisory Panel: a model for determining whether a project is a performance or quality improvement activity or research." Mil Med 175(4): 289-91.[62 Platteborze]
Junod, V. and B. Elger (2010). "Retrospective research: What are the ethical and legal requirements?" Swiss Med Wkly 140: w13041.[63 Junod]
Hansson, M. G. (2010). "Need for a wider view of autonomy in epidemiological research." BMJ 340: c2335.[64 Hansson]
Guta, A., M. G. Wilson, et al. (2010). "Are we asking the right questions? A review of Canadian REB practices in relation to community-based participatory research." J Empir Res Hum Res Ethics 5(2): 35-46.[65 Guta]
Goldberg, M. S. (2010). "The intersection of sound principles of environmental epidemiologic research and ethical guidelines and review: an example from Canada of an environmental case-control study." Rev Environ Health 25(2): 147-60.[66]
Dokholyan, R. S., L. H. Muhlbaier, et al. (2009). "Regulatory and ethical considerations for linking clinical and administrative databases." Am Heart J 157(6): 971-82.[67]
Savel, R. H., E. B. Goldstein, et al. (2009). "Critical care checklists, the Keystone Project, and the Office for Human Research Protections: a case for streamlining the approval process in quality-improvement research." Crit Care Med 37(2): 725-8.[68]
Nerenz, D. R. (2009). "Ethical issues in using data from quality management programs." Eur Spine J 18 Suppl 3: 321-30.[69]
Buchanan, E. A. and E. E. Hvizdak (2009). "Online survey tools: ethical and methodological concerns of human research ethics committees." J Empir Res Hum Res Ethics 4(2): 37-48.[70]
Willison, D. J., C. Emerson, et al. (2008). "Access to medical records for research purposes: varying perceptions across research ethics boards." J Med Ethics 34(4): 308-14.[71]
Reynolds, J., N. Crichton, et al. (2008). "Determining the need for ethical review: a three-stage Delphi study." J Med Ethics 34(12): 889-94.[72]
Miller, F. G. and E. J. Emanuel (2008). "Quality-improvement research and informed consent." N Engl J Med 358(8): 765-7.[73]
Miller, F. G. (2008). "Research on medical records without informed consent." J Law Med Ethics 36(3): 560-6.[74]
Lemaire, F. (2008). "Informed consent and studies of a quality improvement program." JAMA 300(15): 1762; author reply 1762-3.[75]
Hutton, J. L., M. P. Eccles, et al. (2008). "Ethical issues in implementation research: a discussion of the problems in achieving informed consent." Implement Sci 3: 52.[76]
Chaney, E., L. G. Rabuck, et al. (2008). "Human subjects protection issues in QUERI implementation research: QUERI Series." Implement Sci 3: 10.[77]
Lynn, J., M. A. Baily, et al. (2007). "The ethics of using quality improvement methods in health care." Ann Intern Med 146(9): 666-73.[57]
Flicker, S., R. Travers, et al. (2007). "Ethical dilemmas in community-based participatory research: recommendations for institutional review boards." J Urban Health 84(4): 478-93.[78]
Campbell, B., H. Thomson, et al. (2007). "Extracting information from hospital records: what patients think about consent." Qual Saf Health Care 16(6): 404-8.[79]
Baily, M. A., M. Bottrell, et al. (2006). "The ethics of using QI methods to improve health care quality and safety." Hastings Cent Rep 36(4): S1-40.[58]
Ernst, A. A., S. J. Weiss, et al. (2005). "Minimal-risk waiver of informed consent and exception from informed consent (Final Rule) studies at institutional review boards nationwide." Acad Emerg Med 12(11): 1134-7.[80]
Bodenheimer, T., D. M. Young, et al. (2005). "Practice-based research in primary care: facilitator of, or barrier to, practice improvement?" Ann Fam Med 3 Suppl 2: S28-32.[81]
Stimler, C. (2003). "Quality improvement projects: inaction presents the greatest risk." Arch Intern Med 163(21): 2648-9; author reply 2649.[82]
Nerenz, D. R., P. K. Stoltz, et al. (2003). "Quality improvement and the need for IRB review." Qual Manag Health Care 12(3): 159-70.[83]
Lo, B. and M. Groman (2003). "Oversight of quality improvement: focusing on benefits and risks." Arch Intern Med 163(12): 1481-6.[59]
Lindenauer, P. K., E. M. Benjamin, et al. (2002). "The role of the institutional review board in quality improvement: a survey of quality officers, institutional review board chairs, and journal editors." Am J Med 113(7): 575-9.[84]
Hirshon, J. M., S. D. Krugman, et al. (2002). "Variability in institutional review board assessment of minimal-risk research." Acad Emerg Med 9(12): 1417-20.[85]
Doezema, D. and M. Hauswald (2002). "Quality improvement or research: a distinction without a difference?" IRB 24(4): 9-12.[86]
Cassell, J. and A. Young (2002). "Why we should not seek individual informed consent for participation in health services research." J Med Ethics 28(5): 313-7.[87]
Casarett, D., J. H. Karlawish, et al. (2000). "Determining when quality improvement initiatives should be considered research: proposed criteria and potential implications." JAMA 283(17): 2275-80.[60]

Conflict of Interest

We identified 11 publications that dealt with conflict of interest in research, both potential conflict of interest by investigators and potential conflict of interest by IRB members.[13, 88-100] Of the issues we reviewed, this one had the largest body of literature to help inform VA policy. Therefore, we selected it for more detailed review (see Key Question #2).

Payment to Patients and Providers

Payments to patients and payments to health care professionals to enroll patients both are a particular type of conflict of interest. We considered them separate from the other COI articles because they seemed distinct from issues about disclosure in the other COI articles. We identified nine publications that dealt with ethical issues regarding compensating patients to participate in research studies or paying heath care professionals to recruit patients into these studies (Table 4).[15, 101-108] Two of these articles were opinions or commentaries.[103, 107] Four of the articles were descriptive studies about payments to patients. A survey of studies approved in 1997 of 32 "geographically diverse organizations involved in the development, conduct and review of biomedical research" found that 30 (94 percent) paid some participants in clinical studies. About one-third of organizations had written policies or guidelines on payment. Since few written policies exist, standards vary.[108] A follow up study assessed policies on the offering of payment to research participants approved by seven academic and four independent IRBs in 1997. Across studies, there was, in general, no indication that the payment was related to procedures to be performed or the time commitment required to participate in the study. The studies indicated a wide variation in the size of payments, ranging from $5 to $2000, with a median of $155.[104]

Two studies by the same investigator assessed the potential reasons for payments to participants. In the first study, a web-based survey of hundreds of IRB chairpersons and investigators (with a 24 percent response rate) presented six hypothetical research scenarios that varied by the time involved, funding source, and risk. Respondents were asked to select what they considered an appropriate payment from a list of possible figures. The results indicate that individuals consider different factors in determining payment for studies.[109] A related study found that 60 percent, 54 percent, and 42 percent of respondents recommended only a token payment (none or payment only for parking) for studies involving four phone surveys, a one-visit study for DNA collection via buccal swab, and a cancer treatment trial involving 24 visits, meaning that the time spent by the patient vastly exceeded any compensation.[110]

Three publications dealt with the practice of paying healthcare professionals for patient recruitment into clinical trials.[102, 105, 106] The largest of these was a systematic review that searched standard databases through 2006 and identified a small number of original studies: 3 cross sectional surveys, two studies from primary care, and one study from hospital care. The authors could draw no conclusions from their limited evidence base.[111] A second study assessed (from available websites) the policies of 117 IRBs regarding such payments. Only about 25 percent of IRBs had policies about physicians recruiting their own patients for study.[106] The last publication was a commentary about the potential hazards of large payments for patient enrollments.[105]

Table 4. Payment to Patients Articles

Payment to Patients
Brown JS, Schonfeld TL, Gordon BG. "You may have already won..": an examination of the use of lottery payments in research. IRB 2006;28:12-6.[107]
DeRenzo EG. Coercion in the recruitment and retention of human research subjects, pharmaceutical industry payments to physician-investigators, and the moral courage of the IRB. IRB 2000;22:1-5.[103]
Dickert N, Emanuel E, Grady C. Paying research subjects: an analysis of current policies. Ann Intern Med 2002;136:368-73.[108]
Grady C, Dickert N, Jawetz T, Gensler G, Emanuel E. An analysis of U.S. practices of paying research participants. Contemp Clin Trials 2005;26:365-75.[104]
Hall MA, Friedman JY, King NM, Weinfurt KP, Schulman KA, Sugarman J. Commentary: Per capita payments in clinical trials: reasonable costs versus bounty hunting. Acad Med;85:1554-6.[105]
Raftery J, Bryant J, Powell J, Kerr C, Hawker S. Payment to healthcare professionals for patient recruitment to trials: systematic review and qualitative study. Health Technol Assess 2008;12:1-128, iii.[102]
Ripley E, Macrina F, Markowitz M, Gennings C. Who's doing the math? Are we really compensating research participants? J Empir Res Hum Res Ethics 2010;5:57-65.[15]
Ripley E, Macrina F, Markowitz M, Gennings C. Why do we pay? A national survey of investigators and IRB chairpersons. J Empir Res Hum Res Ethics 2010;5:43-56.[101]
Wolf LE. IRB policies regarding finder's fees and role conflicts in recruiting research participants. IRB 2009;31:14-9.[106]

Genetic Studies

We identified eight publications that dealt with potential ethical issues arising from genetic studies that involved the IRB (Table 5).[12, 88, 89, 112-116] One article described a 1995 consensus process for recommendations for informed consent for patients participating in genetic studies.[113] Another described an anonymous survey of IRB chairpersons (22 percent response rate) that found considerable variation in IRB practices regarding informed consent for genetic studies.[115] An in-person survey of Canadian Research Ethic Boards about bio-banks found variability in what was required for the duration of consent.[114] Another study characterized the ethical, legal, and social issues unique to genetic database research.[116] Another publication analyzed the websites of the IRBs from the top 25 NIH funded medical schools,[112] and another presented the findings of a survey of clinical research centers.[12] Finally, two studies categorized as genetics studies also dealt with the topic of conflict of interest and are discussed in that section.[88, 89]

Table 5. Genetic Studies Articles

Genetics
Austin MA, Harding SE, McElroy CE. Monitoring ethical, legal, and social issues in developing population genetic databases. Genet Med 2003;5:451-7.[116]
Clayton EW, Steinberg KK, Khoury MJ, Thomson E, Andrews L, Kahn MJ, Kopelman LM, Weiss JO. Informed consent for genetic research on stored tissue samples. JAMA 1995;274:1786-92.[113]
Gibson E, Brazil K, Coughlin MD, Emerson C, Fournier F, Schwartz L, Szala-Meneok KV, Weisbaum KM, Willison DJ. Who's minding the shop? The role of Canadian research ethics boards in the creation and uses of registries and biobanks. BMC Med Ethics 2008;9:17.[114]
Lipworth W, Kerridge I. Impediments to "T2" research: are ethics really to blame? Am J Bioeth. 2010;10(8):39-40.[89]
Sofaer N, Eyal N. The diverse ethics of translational research. Am J Bioeth. 2010;10(8):19-30.[88]
White MT, Gamm J. Informed consent for research on stored blood and tissue samples: a survey of institutional review board practices. Account Res 2002;9:1-16.[115]
Wolf LE, Bouley TA, McCulloch CE. Genetic research with stored biological materials: ethics and practice. IRB 2010;32:7-18.[12]
Wolf LE, Lo B. Untapped potential: IRB guidance for the ethical research use of stored biological materials. IRB 2004;26:1-8.[112]

Miscellaneous

Eighteen publications were potentially relevant to the IRB's role in maintaining research integrity, but did not fall into one of the existing categories (Table 6).[117-134] These articles represent a mixture of surveys about ethical issues, particularly challenging scenarios that might require special rules (such as practice-based research networks, palliative care, and nursing research) and methods to evaluate the workings of the IRB.

Table 6. Miscellaneous Articles

Miscellaneous
Angell EL, Bryman A, Ashcroft RE, Dixon-Woods M. An analysis of decision letters by research ethics committees: the ethics/scientific quality boundary examined. Qual Saf Health Care 2008;17:131-6.[131]
Barrett R. Strategies for promoting the scientific integrity of nursing research in clinical settings. J Nurses Staff Dev 2010;26:200-5; quiz 260-7.[121]
Campbell EG, Weissman JS, Clarridge B, Yucel R, Causino N, Blumenthal D. Characteristics of medical school faculty members serving on institutional review boards: results of a national survey. Acad Med 2003;78:831-6.[125]
Coleman CH, Bouesseau MC. How do we know that research ethics committees are really working? The neglected role of outcomes assessment in research ethics review. BMC Med Ethics 2008;9:6.[128]
Dixon-Woods M, Angell E, Ashcroft RE, Bryman A. Written work: the social functions of Research Ethics Committee letters. Soc Sci Med 2007;65:792-802.[132]
Kodish E, Stocking C, Ratain MJ, Kohrman A, Siegler M. Ethical issues in phase I oncology research: a comparison of investigators and institutional review board chairpersons. J Clin Oncol 1992;10:1810-6.[122]
Macneil SD, Fernandez CV. Informing research participants of research results: analysis of Canadian university based research ethics board policies. J Med Ethics 2006;32:49-54.[134]
MacNeil SD, Fernandez CV. Attitudes of research ethics board chairs towards disclosure of research results to participants: results of a national survey. J Med Ethics 2007;33:549-53.[133]
Paasche-Orlow MK, Brancati FL. Assessment of medical school institutional review board policies regarding compensation of subjects for research-related injury. Am J Med 2005;118:175-80.[123]
Sacca L. The uncontrolled clinical trial: scientific, ethical, and practical reasons for being. Intern Emerg Med 2010;5:201-4.[120]
Schuppli CA, Fraser D. Factors influencing the effectiveness of research ethics committees. J Med Ethics 2007;33:294-301.[129]
Sirotin N, Wolf LE, Pollack LM, Catania JA, Dolcini MM, Lo B. IRBs and ethically challenging protocols: views of IRB chairs about useful resources. IRB 2010;32:10-9.[119]
Stevens T, Wilde D, Paz S, Ahmedzai SH, Rawson A, Wragg D. Palliative care research protocols: a special case for ethical review? Palliat Med 2003;17:482-90.[124]
Taylor PL. State payer mandates to cover care in US oncology trials: do science and ethics matter? J Natl Cancer Inst 2010;102:376-90.[118]
Weil C, Rooney L, McNeilly P, Cooper K, Borror K, Andreason P. OHRP compliance oversight letters: an update. IRB 2010;32:1-6.[135]
Wichman A, Kalyan DN, Abbott LJ, Wesley R, Sandler AL. Protecting human subjects in the NIH's Intramural Research Program: a draft instrument to evaluate convened meetings of its IRBs. IRB 2006;28:7-10.[130]
Wolf LE, Croughan M, Lo B. The challenges of IRB review and human subjects protections in practice-based research. Med Care 2002;40:521-9.[126]
Wolf LE, Walden JF, Lo B. Human subjects issues and IRB review in practice-based research. Ann Fam Med 2005;3 Suppl 1:S30-7.[127]

KEY QUESTION #2: What is the actual evidence regarding the issue with the largest literature which may inform VA policy? A Detailed Review of Conflict of Interest Studies

Conflict of interest (COI) is increasingly recognized as an important aspect of maintaining public trust in medical research. In 2011, in response to lay media reports of a number of federally funded investigators who failed to disclose millions of dollars in support from companies with a financial interest in the outcome of the research, the NIH released regulations revising its earlier 1995 regulations. Medical journals are requiring increasingly detailed disclosure about potential COI, and the disclosure of COI is one of the primary foci of the recent Institute of Medicine report, "Guidelines We Can Trust." Between 1994 and 2003, 65 of the 77 most-cited clinical trials were financed, partially or completely, with money from industry.[136] Researchers conducting trials for which the findings have potential financial consequences (creating competing interests) are significantly more positive towards the results of their investigations than those without such interests.[137] In addition, studies sponsored by pharmaceutical companies are more likely to have outcomes favorable to these sponsors than investigations receiving other funding, and trials funded by for-profit organizations (companies that may incur financial gain or loss depending on the outcome) were more likely to report positive findings than those supported by not-for-profit organizations.[138, 139] What makes such observations so compelling is that research findings may serve as promotional material and may influence development and contents of practice guideline.[135, 140] In fact, in one study, 87 percent of authors of guidelines had ties with industry that were often not disclosed.[141] IRB members, too, have industry ties, with 36 percent of IRB members disclosing some kind of financial relationship with industry.[93] Of concern, 15.6 percent of IRB members reported that a protocol had been presented in a biased way by an IRB member with industry ties, and 33 percent of IRBs did not require their members to formally disclose relationships with industry.[93]

The evidence contained in the 14 studies reviewed in this section is organized into the following categories:

- Goals of Disclosure
- Who has Policies Around Disclosure
- Persons with Interest That Requires Disclosure
- Parties to Whom Disclosure Must be Made
- Managing Disclosure
- Managing Noncompliance
- Implementing the Policies
- Potential Harms of Disclosure

Many studies contributed evidence to more than one category.

Goals of Disclosure

Investigators used 5 years of data from the NIH Conflict of Interest Notification study to identify six goals of disclosure, particularly when disclosing to potential research subjects. These goals included promoting informed decision making, respecting participants' perceived right to know, establishing or maintaining trust, minimizing risk of legal liability, deterring troubling financial relationships, and protecting research participants' welfare.[94]

In the opinion of these authors, disclosing COI to potential research subjects has three goals:

- promoting autonomy by providing people with information material to making informed decisions about participating in research,
- avoiding legal liability by meeting basic legal or regulatory requirements without hindering research and deterrence, and
- discouraging individuals and institutions from holding conflicts of interest.[142]

A review of the disclosure policies of 120 academic medical centers found that the majority of the institutions' policies were most consistent with the goal of avoiding legal liability.[92]

Another study collected data and feedback from IRB and Conflict of Interest Committee (COIC) officials, individuals with and without health conditions, patients seen in a general medicine primary care clinic, and a multidisciplinary panel of experts and then developed a model disclosure statement. The statement had two versions, one generic and one specific. The generic statement reads:

> "The person leading this medical research study might benefit financially from this study. The Institutional Review Board and a committee at ABC University have reviewed the possibility of financial benefit. They believe that the possible financial benefit to the person leading the research is not likely to affect your safety and/or the scientific quality of the study. If you would like more information, please ask the researchers or the study coordinator." (Page 4)

The specific version of the disclosure statement reads:

> "The person leading this medical research study might benefit financially from this study. Specifically, [insert appropriate description from below]. The Institutional Review Board and a committee at ABC University have reviewed the possibility of financial benefit. They believe that the possible financial benefit to the person leading the research is not likely to affect your safety and/or the scientific quality of the study. If you would like more information, please ask the researchers or the study coordinator" (Page 5.)

The descriptions available for insertion included salary support, money received outside of the study, per capita payments, finders' fees restricted to research uses, unrestricted finders' fees, a researcher or university holding a patent, and a researcher or university owning equity.[96]

A study in which investigators, IRB chairs, and a conflict-of-interest committee (COIC) chairs at ten academic medical centers were interviewed found that 75 percent of investigators (n=8) believed that COI should be disclosed to potential research participants in all circumstances, with half of them believing it should depend on the degree of financial relationship involved. Of the IRB chairs (n=23), 61 percent believed that disclosure should be made in all circumstances, 43 percent believed that it should depend on the degree of financial relationship involved, 9 percent believed it depends on the risk to subjects, and 22 percent responded 'other' (because these data came from analysis of coded transcripts of interviews, respondents could provide more than one coded response for any category; hence percentages may sum to greater than 100 percent and yield apparently conflicting findings). The majority of COIC chairs (n=14) believed disclosure should occur in all circumstances (57 percent of respondents) and depending on the degree of financial relationship involved (50 percent of respondents).

More than half of the investigators identified the rationale for, or benefits of, disclosure as the right to know, making more informed decisions, and/or transparency/honesty; and somewhat fewer than half of the investigators identified liability, the general warning to participants, building trust, public perceptions or "other." Of the IRB chairs, more than half identified more informed decision, and transparency/honesty with fewer than half identifying other benefits, including citing regulations as a benefit. Of the COIC chairs, more than half identified making more informed decisions and building trust, with fewer than half citing the other benefits.

As for the information to be disclosed, more than half of the investigators included the funding source, amount of funding, ties between investigator and sponsor, potential consequences of ties between investigator and sponsor, and "other." Fewer than half thought it necessary to specify that the patient can ask questions. The IRB and COIC chairs answered similarly, except that half (or less) thought potential consequences of ties between investigator and sponsor needed to be reported. The report also summarized beliefs surrounding the timing of the disclosure, with 88 percent of the investigators believing it should be within the informed consent document, compared to 52 percent of the IRB chairs and 29 percent of the COIC chairs.

One fourth of the investigators thought the information should be included in an educational brochure, compared to 4 percent of the IRB chairs and none of the COIC chairs. One fourth of the investigators believed it should be part of the informed consent process, compared to 43 percent of the IRB chairs and COIC chairs. This study documents potentially important differences in the perceived goals of disclosure among these various stakeholders.[97]

Who has Policies around Disclosure?

Conflicts of Interest among Researchers

On October 1, 1995, the Public Health Service and the National Science Foundation declared guidelines surrounding disclosure of COI. The threshold for disclosure of COI was $10,000 in annual income or equity in a relevant company or five percent ownership of such a company. These guidelines gave research institutions discretion in managing conflicts of interest and required that the existence of conflicts of interest that met this threshold be reported to the funding agency before the funds were used.[99]

Lo and colleagues reviewed the COI policies of the 10 medical schools receiving the largest amount of funding from NIH (Baylor College, Columbia University, Harvard, Johns Hopkins, the University of Pennsylvania, University of California at Los Angeles, University of California at San Francisco, University of Washington, Washington University at St. Louis, and Yale University). All required disclosure of financial interests, including stock and stock options and income from salary, honoraria, and consulting fees. Five institutions required disclosure of all financial interest, regardless of the value, whereas the rest followed the federal guidelines and required disclosure only of amounts exceeding $10,000. All ten institutions required disclosures to a university official or committee, but only six institutions required disclosure to the IRB, and only two of these six required disclosure to research subjects.[100]

A national survey of policies on disclosure of COI in biomedical research expanded these data to include responses from medical schools and other research institutions (N=250) that received more than $5 million in total grants annually from the NIH or the National Science Foundation, 47 journals in basic science and clinical medicine, and 16 federal agencies. Of these entities, five medical schools and 10 other research institutions (6 percent of the 250 institutions that responded) reported that they had no policies regarding COI. Among those that did have policies, 91 percent adhered to the federal threshold for disclosure, with 9 percent exceeding (were stricter than) those guidelines. Among the journals, 43 percent (20 journals) reported that they had policies requiring disclosure of COI. Of the 16 federal agencies, four had policies that explicitly addressed COI in extramural research and all but one of the agencies relied primarily on institutional discretion. Within these policies, the specific interests that were required to be disclosed included income (91 percent of policies), equity interest (93 percent), intellectual property (73 percent), finder's fees (1 percent), fiduciary interest only (57 percent), appearance of conflict (66 percent), support of the research (34 percent), and other in-kind support (44 percent). This survey also assessed when, specifically, disclosure was required: Disclosure was required annually or semiannually in 82 percent, upon a material change creating a new potential for conflicts in 76 percent, when a conflict is anticipated in 57 percent, on application for funding in 63 percent, and on award of funding in 9 percent.[99]

Another survey compared COI policies of academic and nonacademic research settings by surveying officials at 199 sites that contributed participants to commercially sponsored phase-3 clinical trials published in JAMA or the New England Journal of Medicine in 2006 and 2007. They found that 97 percent of academic medical centers and 87 percent of nonacademic medical centers followed written COI policies, compared to only 44 percent of outpatient non-academic sites. Within these policies, 49 percent of the institutions used a monetary threshold below which there was no review of investigator's financial relationships; 29 percent of the non-academic medical centers and 16 percent of the non-academic outpatient settings adhered to this policy. This threshold was equal to the NIH threshold in 73 percent of academic medical centers, 68 percent of non-academic medical centers, and 20 percent of non-academic outpatient sites, respectively. Fewer than half of the sites, regardless of type, reported that they reviewed whether per capita payments for conducting research exceeded the reasonable costs of conducting the research.[13]

Conflicts of Interest within an IRB

A study of IRBs from the 121 medical schools that received NIH funding in 2003 found that 74 percent (92/124 one school had 4 IRBs) had written policies that addressed IRB members' COI. Seventy-nine percent of those institutions with written policies defined what constituted a COI: 10 of these required any financial interest to be disclosed, 23 required anything greater than $10,000 to be disclosed, four stated significant financial interests needed to be disclosed (but did not define the threshold), and 14 had no definition of a financial interest.[91]

In 2005, an anonymous survey specifically targeted the IRB chairs who serve at the most research-intensive medical institutions in the US. Out of the 211 respondents (of 296 eligible), 68 percent stated that their IRB has a written policy defining a COI, 22 percent stated that their IRB did not, and 9 percent did not know.[95]

A survey of the policies of academic medical centers was conducted to look specifically for items pertaining to disclosing COI to potential research participants. In this survey, 57 of the 120 academic medical centers (48 percent) mentioned disclosure of COI to potential research subjects. Of these, 58 percent required or suggested verbatim language for the informed consent document. All required disclosure of the study sponsor, but only 38 percent required that the nature of the financial relationship be disclosed. Only 18 percent specified disclosing how funds are allocated, and only 4 percent required notification that the protocol had been reviewed by the COI committee or other administrative body. A few (5 percent) made reference to non-financial interests, and none contained guidelines about disclosing the amount of money involved.[92]

Persons with Interest Requiring Disclosure

Little agreement was seen in surveys on which person or entity was required to disclose a COI. All the "top 10" medical schools required disclosure by full-time and part-time faculty and the investigators' spouses and dependent children.[100] One university extended disclosure to "de facto spouses," parents, siblings, and adult children. Two universities also required disclosure of any "trust, organization, or enterprise" over which the faculty member "exercises a controlling interest." Four policies applied to all research staff and three other policies applied to selected research staff, generally those with "responsibility for the design, conduct, and reporting of research." Four policies also applied to trainees.[100]

In the survey of the policies of 235 medical schools and other research entities, all investigators were required to disclose, but "family" was expanded to include not only the spouse or partner (89 percent) and minor or dependent child (89 percent), but also another household member (32 percent), adult child (23 percent), parent (22 percent), grandchild (6 percent), another relative (15 percent), unspecified family (2 percent) and a trust (6 percent).[99]

Among policies specific to IRBs, 99 percent referred to all IRB members, and one policy referred only to IRB chairs. In addition, 14 percent of policies extended to IRB staff, 20 percent of policies specified ad hoc reviewers and consultants, and only 4 percent extended to guests.[91]

In the study that compared academic and non-academic research sites, 100 percent of the academic medical centers required investigators to report financial relationships in clinical research, whereas 96 percent of the non-academic medical centers and 90 percent of the non-academic outpatient settings required this disclosure. Non-employee investigators were also covered, with the institution reviewing the financial relationships of non-employee investigators in 90 percent of the academic medical centers, 83 percent of the non-academic medical centers, and 67 percent of the non-academic outpatient settings. If the institution did not review these non-employee relationships, another institution or office reviewed them in 100 percent of the academic medical centers, 70 percent of the non-academic medical centers, and 33 percent of the non-academic outpatient settings.[13]

Parties to Whom Disclosure Must be Made

Conflicts of Interest among Researchers

The reviewed studies often failed to specify the party to whom the disclosure must be made. The study of the policies of the 10 medical schools receiving the largest amount of funding from the NIH found that all 10 required that disclosure of COI be made to a university committee or official "who would either approve the disclosed financial arrangements or ensure that steps were taken to manage, reduce, or eliminate the conflict of interest." Six of those institutions also required that disclosure of financial interests be made to the IRB. Two of these institutions also required disclosure to be made to research participants. Four institutions required that disclosure be made in presentations and published articles.[100]

When the survey was expanded to include a larger number of institutions, responses revealed that 100 percent of the medical schools surveyed (235/235) required initial disclosure to some party within the institution, with only one percent requiring initial disclosure to be made to the IRB, eight percent to the funding agency or sponsor, one percent to research subjects, and seven percent to journals. One school also stipulated that disclosure be made to collaborating researchers.[99]

Interestingly, a separate study that surveyed academic medical centers, explicitly searching for information about disclosing COI to potential research subjects, 48 percent of their policies mentioned such disclosure as a possible strategy for managing conflicts.[92]

In the study comparing academic and non-academic settings, the IRB had a role in review of investigators' financial relationships in clinical research in 74 percent of academic medical centers, 73 percent of non-academic medical centers, and 74 percent of non-academic outpatient settings. Other persons or groups with a role in review of investigators financial relationships in clinical research included the COI committee (45 percent, 9 percent, 1 percent respectively); compliance department (5 percent, 2 percent, 0.4 percent); legal department (2 percent, 3 percent, 0.4 percent); research office, department, or committee (4 percent, 8 percent, 1 percent); sponsor (1 percent, 1 percent, 7 percent); board (1 percent, 0, 1 percent); key individual (11 percent, 6 percent, 3 percent); other (10 percent, 3 percent, 1 percent); or no other review (3 percent, 7 percent, 10 percent).[13]

A national survey of five groups of research stakeholders, including researchers, research officials, bioethicists, editors of journals, and federal agency officials, questioned them about requirements for disclosure of COI to IRBs, research subjects, journals, and funding agencies. Overall, all of these stakeholders gave some level of support to disclosure to IRBs, research subjects, journals, and funding agencies. However, only the bioethicists were *strongly* supportive of including research participants.[98]

Conflicts of Interest within an IRB

When IRB chairs were surveyed, 62 percent responded that their IRB members reported their industry relationships to the IRB chair, 76 percent of respondents reported to the entire IRB, 53 percent of respondents reported to a group or individual within the organization but separate from the IRB, 7 percent reported to an entity external to the IRB and the institution that it serves, and 2 percent reported to an unnamed 'other.'[95]

Managing Disclosure

Within the policies of the 235 medical schools and other research institutions, disclosure was managed by divestment of interest (62 percent), withdrawal of the investigator from the project (61 percent), disclosure to the IRB or research participants (0 percent), disclosure to the funding agency or sponsor (43 percent), disclosure to journals (2 percent), disclosure to collaborating researchers (1 percent), a modification of research plan (59 percent), monitoring of the project (66 percent), requiring additional peer review (7 percent), or public disclosure (59 percent). Only one of the institutions had a mandatory management method, with the remainder relying on a discretionary management method.[99]

When IRB chairs were surveyed regarding what occurred following the disclosure of a conflict of interest, management was decided by the IRB chair in 27 percent of the institutions, the entire IRB in 31 percent, a group or individual within the organization but separate from the IRB in 16 percent, a written policy in 13 percent, and the IRB member in 13 percent.[95]

Prohibited Interests

Absolute prohibitions on particular COI were less common. One of the 'top 10' institutions prohibits faculty from having stock-options, consulting agreements, and decision-making positions that involved a company sponsoring a study in which the faculty member is participating. Another institution prohibited trading in stock or stock options in the company sponsoring the research or selling the product or device being investigated. Two other institutions did not prohibit but did not allow faculty to participate in research if they had a 'significant' financial interest "in the company owning or licensing the product or device being studied."[100]

When comparing academic to nonacademic research settings, 30 percent of academic medical centers, 33 percent of non-academic medical centers, and 5 percent of non-academic outpatient settings prohibited consulting; 52 percent, 44 percent, and 82 percent prohibited equity; 30 percent, 33 percent, and 36 percent prohibited per capita payments; and 70 percent, 59 percent, and 36 percent had unspecified 'other' prohibitions.

Monitoring Compliance

No studies were identified that described how compliance was monitored.

Managing Noncompliance

Methods of managing non-compliance with a COI policy varied across institutions. In a survey of IRB policies, only 4 of 92 (four percent), discussed what occurs when members failed to comply with the COI policies of their own IRB. One described such actions as reporting the non-compliance to institutional officials with possible removal from the IRB, revocation of the member's institutional appointment, and potential sanctions from federal oversight agencies. The others mentioned only removal from the IRB.[91]

When looking at the policies of 235 medical schools and other research entities, the penalty for non-disclosure of COI was termination (46 percent); suspension (20 percent); salary modification (12 percent); non-financial modification, e.g., loss of research space (12 percent); reprimand (28 percent); disqualification from future grant applications (19 percent); notification of funding agency, journal, or both of nondisclosure (42 percent); removal of investigator from project (5 percent); unspecified or nonspecific penalty (46 percent); mandatory penalty (0); or discretionary penalty (100 percent).[99]

Implementing the Policies

The majority of these studies assessed the policies in place, most likely assuming that the policy was enforced. Two of the studies assessed how well the policies were implemented when a COI was identified. In a study of a random sample of 893 IRB members, 78 reported that in the previous year, their IRB reviewed at least one protocol for a study sponsored by a company with which they had a relationship, or a competitor of that company. Of these IRB members, 58 percent always disclosed the relationship to an IRB official, 8 percent sometimes did, 12 percent rarely did and 23 percent never did. Of the 62 who were voting members of their IRBs (not all IRB members are voting members), 65 percent reported that they never voted on a protocol for which they had a financial interest, 5 percent rarely did, 11 percent sometimes did, and 19 percent always did.[93]

An anonymous survey asked IRB chairs, "in hindsight, over the last year, how confident are you that your IRB's processes and procedures provided the appropriate level of disclosure for every study in which a member-industry relationship existed?" Most were moderately confident (41.5 percent vs. 38.7 percent very confident, 15.1 percent not very confident and 4.1 percent not at all confident). In addition, they were asked to recall what happened when a member had a conflict of interest with industry. For example, 63.8 percent answered that the member always left the room when the protocol was under consideration, 10.6 percent answered that the member 'never' left the room, 10.6 percent answered that the member 'rarely' left, and 14.9 percent answered that the member 'usually' left the room. When asked if that member fully participated in the general discussion, 63 percent answered 'never,' 21.7 percent 'rarely,' 8.7 percent 'usually,' and 6.5 percent 'always.' Regarding whether the member voted on the protocol, 100 percent answered 'never.' They were also asked to rate their confidence that the IRB managed conflicts correctly in every case. Two percent were 'not at all confident,' two percent were 'not very confident,' 62 percent were 'moderately confident,' and 34 percent were 'very confident.'[95]

Potential Harms of Disclosure

A study for which investigators, IRB chairs, and COIC chairs of ten academic medical centers were interviewed elicited some of the negative effects or barriers to disclosing COI, at least with respect to disclosure to potential research subjects. These barriers included the belief that disclosure "might affect enrollment of participants" (believed by 63 percent (5/8) of investigators, 78 percent (18/23) of IRB chairs, and 79 percent (11/14) of COIC chairs); that disclosure "breaks down trust" (63 percent, 26 percent, and 21 percent, respectively), that disclosure lengthens the informed consent document (38 percent, 26 percent, and 29 percent, respectively); that disclosure lengthens the informed consent process (38 percent, 9 percent, and 0 percent, respectively); that disclosure is unnecessary (25 percent, 0 percent, seven percent, respectively); that disclosure violates issues of investigator privacy (25 percent, 22 percent, and 29 percent, respectively) and that COI are too difficult for research participants to understand (25 percent, 43 percent, and 71 percent, respectively). Some of those surveyed believed there were additional issues, not specified: 62 percent of the investigators, 35 percent of the IRB chairs, and 14 percent of the COIC chairs. Some of those interviewed believed there were no negative effects or barriers to disclosure: 13 percent of the investigators, 4 percent of the IRB chairs, and 29 percent of the COIC chairs.[97]

SUMMARY AND DISCUSSION

Key Question #1

Our search revealed that the largest number of published studies pertaining to IRBs deal with the challenges of getting IRB approval for multi-site research studies and defining when quality improvement initiatives are considered research (these two topics account for 60 percent of the articles we identified). The VA has recently implemented national policies in both of these areas, designed to reduce complexity and uncertainty for researchers while maintaining appropriate safeguards for research participants.

Of the remaining studies, the next most common topic of study was COI, which thus became the focus of Key Question #2. A modest number of studies assessed payments to providers or patients for participating in research; payment policies varied widely across these studies and little relationship was identified between the time expected for patient involvement and the payment.

We also identified a modest number of published studies about the ethics of genetic studies, which is perhaps surprising given the degree of interest in the topic in both professional and lay audiences.

Key Question #2

With regard to COI, we identified a modest number of published studies, almost all of them descriptive and some with substantial limitations (such as low survey response rates or geographic restriction of the sample to a small number of sites). There literature on investigator COI is much richer than that on IRB member COI. Nevertheless, the available evidence indicates potentially worrisome variation in practice across sites. Variation exists in four domains:

1. Who needs to disclose?
   Which members of the research project need to provide COI disclosures? This group could include principal investigator(s), co-investigators, research assistants, and other research staff.
2. What needs to be disclosed?
   This category includes direct financial interests, but also indirect financial support such as support for travel to attend meetings or non-financial conflicts.
3. How distant a relationship may an individual have with an investigator and still be required to disclose COI? How many people in the investigator's family are included in the need for disclosure?
   This group nearly always includes a spouse, but could also include children, parents, siblings, or other extended family members.
4. To whom does the information need to be disclosed? The recipient can range from a specific official or committee within the institution's IRB to research participants.

The challenges raised by each of these domains is that the options within each can multiply quickly, as can be seen in the following chart, using only a few simple categories for who, what, and how distant.

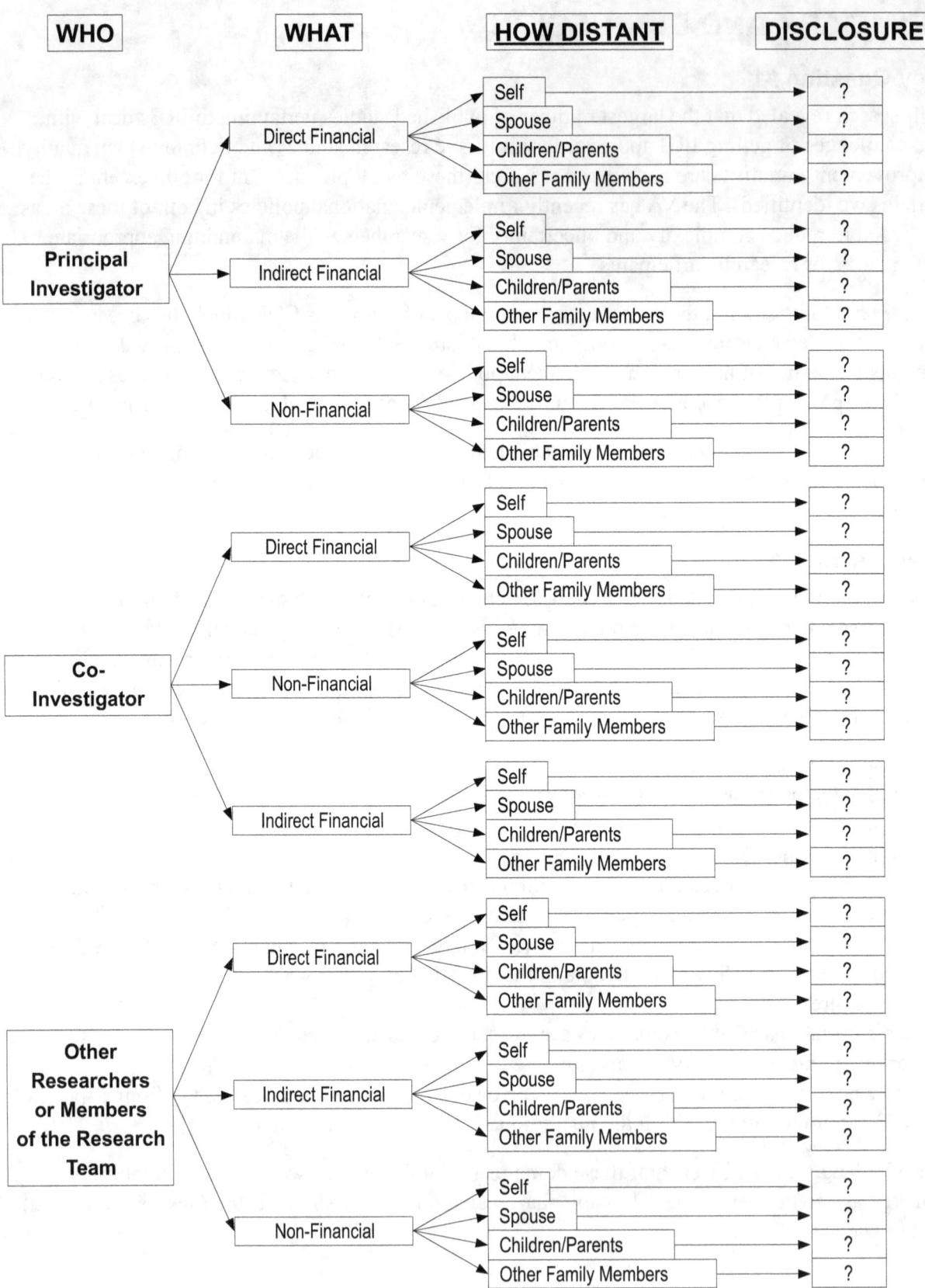

Using only these simple categories provides 36 different ways that institutions can vary in their financial COI policies, without even accounting for the entity to whom should disclosure be made, the thresholds used for many kinds of financial disclosures, and variability in those thresholds ($5,000-$10,000, etc.). Some of the categories are probably clearly not relevant, such as disclosing the non-financial interests of the children/parents of other researchers, whereas others are likely considered mandatory procedures by all academic institutions, such as disclosing direct financial conflicts for the principle investigator of a study. Between these extremes lies much room for variation.

Most of the studies have described variations in policies regarding who and what should be disclosed. The literature on how conflict and non-compliance are managed is particularly thin.

LIMITATIONS

The main limitation of this review is the identification of the primary literature. This topic is not one easily searched with MeSH or title terms, unlike more typical topics of systematic reviews such as randomized trials for the efficacy of pharmaceuticals. Although our initial search was intentionally broad and identified more than 4,000 titles, we may have missed some relevant, original studies. During peer review, a number of additional articles or searches were suggested, but pursuing these did not yield additional research articles. The second limitation is the aggregate limitation in the studies we did identify. Many suffered from poor response rates or limited populations, and drawing broad generalizable conclusions is challenging, beyond the general conclusion of variability in certain domains.

RECOMMENDATIONS FOR FUTURE RESEARCH

Maintaining high ethical standards of conduct in research, both for the investigator and for IRBs, is a high prority for VA, and not one where VA can or should merely react to problems when they are identified. Rather, VA should aim that research conducted at all VA insitutions is held to the same high standard, much as it has done with clinical care over the past 15 years. To do so, VA should:

1. Conduct a descriptive study of current COI practices for investigators and IRB members at all VA facilities,
2. Use this information to determine which areas of current practices have unjustifiable levels of variation across sites,
3. Convene stakeholders to determine best practices for these processes,
4. Create VA-wide policy about these practices, and
5. Monitor implementation across facilities.

As an example, right now it is unknown whether VA facilities vary across the four dimensions of "who should disclose," "what to disclose," "how distant must an individual be related to an investigator to avoid disclosure," and "to whom should COI be disclosed." VA facilities may vary, possibly greatly, in these dimensions. VA has striven to provide, and patients have come to expect, one high standard of clinical care no matter which VA facility they visit. It is unreasonable for Veterans to expect differing ethical standards of research across VA facilities.

Research-informed policy can ensure that COI disclosure be made as standard as clinical care, while allowing local flexibility when it is justified. Implicit in this statement is that defining standard COI policies, while a necessary condition, is not sufficient. Monitoring implementation is critical. AAHRPP has attempted to institute a common standard across VA facilities (at least those that are accredited) with response to a single disclosure threshold, disclosure from all individuals involved in the research, and management plans. One challenge is as a government agency VA must follow the government-wide ethics regulations that state federal employees may not have financial interests that relate to their work. All VA IRBs, that are accredited, have conflict of interest policies.

After this uniformity is accomplished, the next step will be to try and provide national VA guidelines on managing COI for individuals (investigators) and IRBs. While preservation of local autonomy is important for providing insitutions with the flexibility they need, some system-wide principles would be useful to help local sites inform COI management decisions. Non-financial COI will also need to be addressed at some point. Given the current imprecision with which non-financial conflicts are defined, the VA would best defer this topic until a greater degree of consensus is reached in the scientific community on how non-financial conflicts are defined.

Lastly, since many VA insitutions that conduct research have university affiliates, a potential complicating factor is the lack of harmony between VA COI and that of these university affliates.

REFERENCES

1. Germany (Territory under Allied occupation 1945- U. S. Zone) Military Tribunals. [from old catalog], *Trials of war criminals before the Nuernberg Military Tribunals under Control Council law no. 10*. 1949, Washington,: U. S. Govt. Print. Off. 15 v.

2. Association, W.M., *Declaration of Helsinki, 5th (South Africa) amendment.* 2000.

3. Beecher, H.K., *Ethics and clinical research.* N Engl J Med, 1966. 274(24): p. 1354-60.

4. The National Commission for the Protection of Human Subjects of Biomedical and Behavioral Research, *The Belmont Report: Ethical Principles and Guidelines for the Protection of Human Subjects of Research*, E. Department of Health, and Welfare, Editor. 1979: Washington, D.C.

5. *Memorandum of the Surgeon General William H. Stewart to the Heads of Institutions Conducting Research with Public Health Grants*, USPHS, Editor. 1966.

6. Lo, B., M.J. Field, and Institute of Medicine (U.S.). Committee on Conflict of Interest in Medical Research Education and Practice., *Conflict of interest in medical research, education, and practice*. 2009, Washington, D.C.: National Academies Press. xxi, 414 p.

7. Bekelman, J.E., Y. Li, and C.P. Gross, *Scope and impact of financial conflicts of interest in biomedical research.* JAMA, 2003. 289(4): p. 454-65.

8. Institute of Medicine, *Conflict of Interest in Medical Research, Education, and Practice*, B. Lo and M.J. Field, Editors: Washington, D.C.

9. Cho, M.K., et al., *Policies on faculty conflicts of interst at US universities.* JAMA, 2000. 284(17): p. 2203-8.

10. Boyd, E.A., S. Lipton, and L.A. Bero, *Implementation of financial disclosure policies to manage conflicts of interest.* Health Aff, 2004. 23(2): p. 206-14.

11. Boyd, E.A. and L.A. Bero, *Defining financial conflicts and managing research relationships: An analysis of university conflict of interest committee decisions.* Sci Eng Ethics, 2007. 13: p. 415-435.

12. Wolf, L.E., T.A. Bouley, and C.E. McCulloch, *Genetic research with stored biological materials: ethics and practice.* IRB, 2010. 32(2): p. 7-18.

13. Weinfurt, K.P., et al., *Oversight of financial conflicts of interest in commercially sponsored research in academic and nonacademic settings.* J Gen Intern Med, 2010. 25(5): p. 460-4.

14. Taylor, H.A., et al., *The ethical review of health care quality improvement initiatives: findings from the field.* Issue Brief (Commonw Fund), 2010. 95: p. 1-12.

15. Ripley, E., et al., *Who's doing the math? Are we really compensating research participants?* J Empir Res Hum Res Ethics, 2010. 5(3): p. 57-65.

16. Angell, E., et al., *Consistency in decision making by research ethics committees: a controlled comparison.* J Med Ethics, 2006. 32(11): p. 662-4.

17. Blustein, J., et al., *Notes from the field: jumpstarting the IRB approval process in multicenter studies.* Health Serv Res, 2007. 42(4): p. 1773-82.

18. Burman, W., et al., *The effects of local review on informed consent documents from a multicenter clinical trials consortium.* Control Clin Trials, 2003. 24(3): p. 245-55.

19. Burman, W.J., et al., *Breaking the camel's back: multicenter clinical trials and local institutional review boards.* Ann Intern Med, 2001. 134(2): p. 152-7.

20. Christie, D.R., G.S. Gabriel, and K. Dear, *Adverse effects of a multicentre system for ethics approval on the progress of a prospective multicentre trial of cancer treatment: how many patients die waiting?* Intern Med J, 2007. 37(10): p. 680-6.

21. Dilts, D.M. and A.B. Sandler, *Invisible barriers to clinical trials: the impact of structural, infrastructural, and procedural barriers to opening oncology clinical trials.* J Clin Oncol, 2006. 24(28): p. 4545-52.

22. Dyrbye, L.N., et al., *Medical education research and IRB review: an analysis and comparison of the IRB review process at six institutions.* Acad Med, 2007. 82(7): p. 654-60.

23. Dziak, K., et al., *Variations among Institutional Review Board reviews in a multisite health services research study.* Health Serv Res, 2005. 40(1): p. 279-90.

24. Edwards, S.J., T. Stone, and T. Swift, *Differences between research ethics committees.* Int J Technol Assess Health Care, 2007. 23(1): p. 17-23.

25. Elwyn, G., et al., *Ethics and research governance in a multicentre study: add 150 days to your study protocol.* BMJ, 2005. 330(7495): p. 847.

26. Enzle, M.E. and R. Schmaltz, *Ethics review of multi-centre clinical trials in Canada.* Health Law Rev, 2005. 13(2-3): p. 51-7.

27. Ezzat, H., et al., *Ethics review as a component of institutional approval for a multicentre continuous quality improvement project: the investigator's perspective.* BMC Health Serv Res, 2010. 10: p. 223.

28. Gold, J.L. and C.S. Dewa, *Institutional review boards and multisite studies in health services research: is there a better way?* Health Serv Res, 2005. 40(1): p. 291-307.

29. Green, L.A., et al., *Impact of institutional review board practice variation on observational health services research.* Health Serv Res, 2006. 41(1): p. 214-30.

30. Greene, S.M. and A.M. Geiger, *A review finds that multicenter studies face substantial challenges but strategies exist to achieve Institutional Review Board approval.* J Clin Epidemiol, 2006. 59(8): p. 784-90.

31. Greene, S.M., et al., *Impact of IRB requirements on a multicenter survey of prophylactic mastectomy outcomes.* Ann Epidemiol, 2006. 16(4): p. 275-8.

32. Helfand, B.T., et al., *Variation in institutional review board responses to a standard protocol for a multicenter randomized, controlled surgical trial.* J Urol, 2009. 181(6): p. 2674-9.

33. Hicks, S.C., et al., *A case study evaluation of ethics review systems for multicentre clinical trials.* Med J Aust, 2009. 191(5): p. 280-2.

34. Koski, G., et al., *Cooperative research ethics review boards: a win-win solution?* IRB, 2005. 27(3): p. 1-7.

35. McWilliams, R., et al., *Problematic variation in local institutional review of a multicenter genetic epidemiology study.* JAMA, 2003. 290(3): p. 360-6.

36. Menikoff, J., *The paradoxical problem with multiple-IRB review.* N Engl J Med, 2010. 363(17): p. 1591-3.

37. Newgard, C.D., et al., *Institutional variability in a minimal risk, population-based study: recognizing policy barriers to health services research.* Health Serv Res, 2005. 40(4): p. 1247-58.

38. Olver, I.N., *A case study evaluation of ethics review systems for multicentre clinical trials.* Med J Aust, 2010. 192(5): p. 293.

39. Pogorzelska, M., et al., *Changes in the institutional review board submission process for multicenter research over 6 years.* Nurs Outlook, 2010. 58(4): p. 181-7.

40. Racine, E., E. Bell, and C. Deslauriers, *Canadian research ethics boards and multisite research: experiences from two minimal-risk studies.* IRB, 2010. 32(3): p. 12-8.

41. Ravina, B., et al., *Local institutional review board (IRB) review of a multicenter trial: local costs without local context.* Ann Neurol, 2010. 67(2): p. 258-60.

42. Rikkert, M.G., et al., *The practice of obtaining approval from medical research ethics committees: a comparison within 12 European countries for a descriptive study on acetylcholinesterase inhibitors in Alzheimer's dementia.* Eur J Neurol, 2005. 12(3): p. 212-7.

43. Rose, C.D., *Local vs central institutional review boards for multicenter studies.* JAMA, 2003. 290(16): p. 2126; author reply 2126-7.

44. Saginur, R., et al., *Ontario Cancer Research Ethics Board: lessons learned from developing a multicenter regional institutional review board.* J Clin Oncol, 2008. 26(9): p. 1479-82.

45. Sarson-Lawrence, M., et al., *Trust and confidence: towards mutual acceptance of ethics committee approval of multicentre studies.* Intern Med J, 2004. 34(11): p. 598-603.

46. Shelby-James, T., M.R. Agar, and D.C. Currow, *A case study evaluation of ethics review systems for multicentre clinical trials.* Med J Aust, 2010. 192(5): p. 292.

47. Sherwood, M.L., et al., *Unique challenges of obtaining regulatory approval for a multicenter protocol to study the genetics of RRP and suggested remedies.* Otolaryngol Head Neck Surg, 2006. 135(2): p. 189-96.

48. Silverman, H., S.C. Hull, and J. Sugarman, *Variability among institutional review boards' decisions within the context of a multicenter trial.* Crit Care Med, 2001. 29(2): p. 235-41.

49. Stair, T.O., et al., *Variation in institutional review board responses to a standard protocol for a multicenter clinical trial.* Acad Emerg Med, 2001. 8(6): p. 636-41.

50. Stark, A.R., J.E. Tyson, and P.L. Hibberd, *Variation among institutional review boards in evaluating the design of a multicenter randomized trial.* J Perinatol, 2010. 30(3): p. 163-9.

51. Tully, J., et al., *The new system of review by multicentre research ethics committees: prospective study.* BMJ, 2000. 320(7243): p. 1179-82.

52. Vick, C.C., et al., *Variation in Institutional Review processes for a multisite observational study.* Am J Surg, 2005. 190(5): p. 805-9.

53. Wagner, T.H., et al., *The cost of operating institutional review boards (IRBs).* Acad Med, 2003. 78(6): p. 638-44.

54. Wagner, T.H., A.M. Cruz, and G.L. Chadwick, *Economies of scale in institutional review boards.* Med Care, 2004. 42(8): p. 817-23.

55. Wagner, T.H., et al., *Costs and benefits of the national cancer institute central institutional review board.* J Clin Oncol, 2010. 28(4): p. 662-6.

56. Yawn, B.P., et al., *Practice-based research network studies and institutional review boards: two new issues.* J Am Board Fam Med, 2009. 22(4): p. 453-60.

57. Lynn, J., et al., *The ethics of using quality improvement methods in health care.* Ann Intern Med, 2007. 146(9): p. 666-73.

58. Baily, M.A., et al., *The ethics of using QI methods to improve health care quality and safety.* Hastings Cent Rep, 2006. 36(4): p. S1-40.

59. Lo, B. and M. Groman, *Oversight of quality improvement: focusing on benefits and risks.* Arch Intern Med, 2003. 163(12): p. 1481-6.

60. Casarett, D., J.H. Karlawish, and J. Sugarman, *Determining when quality improvement initiatives should be considered research: proposed criteria and potential implications.* JAMA, 2000. 283(17): p. 2275-80.

61. Baily, M.A., *Harming through protection?* N Engl J Med, 2008. 358(8): p. 768--9.

62. Platteborze, L.S., et al., *Performance Improvement/Research Advisory Panel: a model for determining whether a project is a performance or quality improvement activity or research.* Mil Med, 2010. 175(4): p. 289-91.

63. Junod, V. and B. Elger, *Retrospective research: What are the ethical and legal requirements?* Swiss Med Wkly, 2010. 140: p. w13041.

64. Hansson, M.G., *Need for a wider view of autonomy in epidemiological research.* BMJ, 2010. 340: p. c2335.

65. Guta, A., et al., *Are we asking the right questions? A review of Canadian REB practices in relation to community-based participatory research.* J Empir Res Hum Res Ethics, 2010. 5(2): p. 35-46.

66. Goldberg, M.S., *The intersection of sound principles of environmental epidemiologic research and ethical guidelines and review: an example from Canada of an environmental case-control study.* Rev Environ Health, 2010. 25(2): p. 147-60.

67. Dokholyan, R.S., et al., *Regulatory and ethical considerations for linking clinical and administrative databases.* Am Heart J, 2009. 157(6): p. 971-82.

68. Savel, R.H., E.B. Goldstein, and M.A. Gropper, *Critical care checklists, the Keystone Project, and the Office for Human Research Protections: a case for streamlining the approval process in quality-improvement research.* Crit Care Med, 2009. 37(2): p. 725-8.

69. Nerenz, D.R., *Ethical issues in using data from quality management programs.* Eur Spine J, 2009. 18 Suppl 3: p. 321-30.

70. Buchanan, E.A. and E.E. Hvizdak, *Online survey tools: ethical and methodological concerns of human research ethics committees.* J Empir Res Hum Res Ethics, 2009. 4(2): p. 37-48.

71. Willison, D.J., et al., *Access to medical records for research purposes: varying perceptions across research ethics boards.* J Med Ethics, 2008. 34(4): p. 308-14.

72. Reynolds, J., et al., *Determining the need for ethical review: a three-stage Delphi study.* J Med Ethics, 2008. 34(12): p. 889-94.

73. Miller, F.G. and E.J. Emanuel, *Quality-improvement research and informed consent.* N Engl J Med, 2008. 358(8): p. 765-7.

74. Miller, F.G., *Research on medical records without informed consent.* J Law Med Ethics, 2008. 36(3): p. 560-6.

75. Lemaire, F., *Informed consent and studies of a quality improvement program.* JAMA, 2008. 300(15): p. 1762; author reply 1762-3.

76. Hutton, J.L., M.P. Eccles, and J.M. Grimshaw, *Ethical issues in implementation research: a discussion of the problems in achieving informed consent.* Implement Sci, 2008. 3: p. 52.

77. Chaney, E., et al., *Human subjects protection issues in QUERI implementation research: QUERI Series.* Implement Sci, 2008. 3: p. 10.

78. Flicker, S., et al., *Ethical dilemmas in community-based participatory research: recommendations for institutional review boards.* J Urban Health, 2007. 84(4): p. 478-93.

79. Campbell, B., et al., *Extracting information from hospital records: what patients think about consent.* Qual Saf Health Care, 2007. 16(6): p. 404-8.

80. Ernst, A.A., et al., *Minimal-risk waiver of informed consent and exception from informed consent (Final Rule) studies at institutional review boards nationwide.* Acad Emerg Med, 2005. 12(11): p. 1134-7.

81. Bodenheimer, T., et al., *Practice-based research in primary care: facilitator of, or barrier to, practice improvement?* Ann Fam Med, 2005. 3 Suppl 2: p. S28-32.

82. Stimler, C., *Quality improvement projects: inaction presents the greatest risk.* Arch Intern Med, 2003. 163(21): p. 2648-9; author reply 2649.

83. Nerenz, D.R., P.K. Stoltz, and J. Jordan, *Quality improvement and the need for IRB review.* Qual Manag Health Care, 2003. 12(3): p. 159-70.

84. Lindenauer, P.K., et al., *The role of the institutional review board in quality improvement: a survey of quality officers, institutional review board chairs, and journal editors.* Am J Med, 2002. 113(7): p. 575-9.

85. Hirshon, J.M., et al., *Variability in institutional review board assessment of minimal-risk research.* Acad Emerg Med, 2002. 9(12): p. 1417-20.

86. Doezema, D. and M. Hauswald, *Quality improvement or research: a distinction without a difference?* IRB, 2002. 24(4): p. 9-12.

87. Cassell, J. and A. Young, *Why we should not seek individual informed consent for participation in health services research.* J Med Ethics, 2002. 28(5): p. 313-7.

88. Sofaer, N. and N. Eyal, *The diverse ethics of translational research.* Am J Bioeth, 2010. 10(8): p. 19-30.

89. Lipworth, W. and I. Kerridge, *Impediments to "T2" research: are ethics really to blame?* Am J Bioeth, 2010. 10(8): p. 39-40.

90. Kachuck, N.J., *Managing conflicts of interest and commitment: academic medicine and the physician's progress.* J Med Ethics. 37(1): p. 2-5.

91. Wolf, L.E. and J. Zandecki, *Conflicts of interest in research: how IRBs address their own conflicts.* IRB, 2007. 29(1): p. 6-12.

92. Weinfurt, K.P., et al., *Policies of academic medical centers for disclosing financial conflicts of interest to potential research participants.* Acad Med, 2006. 81(2): p. 113-8.

93. Campbell, E.G., et al., *Financial relationships between institutional review board members and industry.* N Engl J Med, 2006. 355(22): p. 2321-9.

94. Weinfurt, K.P., et al., *Disclosure of financial relationships to participants in clinical research.* N Engl J Med, 2009. 361(9): p. 916-21.

95. Vogeli, C., G. Koski, and E.G. Campbell, *Policies and management of conflicts of interest within medical research institutional review boards: results of a national study.* Acad Med, 2009. 84(4): p. 488-94.

96. Weinfurt, K.P., et al., *Developing model language for disclosing financial interests to potential clinical research participants.* IRB, 2007. 29(1): p. 1-5.

97. Weinfurt, K.P., et al., *Disclosing conflicts of interest in clinical research: views of institutional review boards, conflict of interest committees, and investigators.* J Law Med Ethics, 2006. 34(3): p. 581-91, 481.

98. Brody, B.A., et al., *Expanding disclosure of conflicts of interest: the views of stakeholders.* IRB, 2003. 25(1): p. 1-8.

99. McCrary, S.V., et al., *A national survey of policies on disclosure of conflicts of interest in biomedical research.* N Engl J Med, 2000. 343(22): p. 1621-6.

100. Lo, B., L.E. Wolf, and A. Berkeley, *Conflict-of-interest policies for investigators in clinical trials.* N Engl J Med, 2000. 343(22): p. 1616-20.

101. Ripley, E., et al., *Why do we pay? A national survey of investigators and IRB chairpersons.* J Empir Res Hum Res Ethics, 2010. 5(3): p. 43-56.

102. Raftery, J., et al., *Payment to healthcare professionals for patient recruitment to trials: systematic review and qualitative study.* Health Technol Assess, 2008. 12(10): p. 1-128, iii.

103. DeRenzo, E.G., *Coercion in the recruitment and retention of human research subjects, pharmaceutical industry payments to physician-investigators, and the moral courage of the IRB.* IRB, 2000. 22(2): p. 1-5.

104. Grady, C., et al., *An analysis of U.S. practices of paying research participants.* Contemp Clin Trials, 2005. 26(3): p. 365-75.

105. Hall, M.A., et al., *Commentary: Per capita payments in clinical trials: reasonable costs versus bounty hunting.* Acad Med. 85(10): p. 1554-6.

106. Wolf, L.E., *IRB policies regarding finder's fees and role conflicts in recruiting research participants.* IRB, 2009. 31(1): p. 14-9.

107. Brown, J.S., T.L. Schonfeld, and B.G. Gordon, *"You may have already won..": an examination of the use of lottery payments in research.* IRB, 2006. 28(1): p. 12-6.

108. Dickert, N., E. Emanuel, and C. Grady, *Paying research subjects: an analysis of current policies.* Ann Intern Med, 2002. 136(5): p. 368-73.

109. Ripley, E., et al., *Why do we pay? A national survey of investigators and IRB chairpersons.* J Empir Res Hum Res Ethics. 5(3): p. 43-56.

110. Millum, J. and J. Menikoff, *Streamlining ethical review.* Ann Intern Med, 2010. 153(10): p. 655-7.

111. Eastman, N., B. Philips, and A. Rhodes, *Triaging for adult critical care in the event of overwhelming need.* Intensive Care Med, 2010. 36(6): p. 1076-82.

112. Wolf, L.E. and B. Lo, *Untapped potential: IRB guidance for the ethical research use of stored biological materials.* IRB, 2004. 26(4): p. 1-8.

113. Clayton, E.W., et al., *Informed consent for genetic research on stored tissue samples.* JAMA, 1995. 274(22): p. 1786-92.

114. Gibson, E., et al., *Who's minding the shop? The role of Canadian research ethics boards in the creation and uses of registries and biobanks.* BMC Med Ethics, 2008. 9: p. 17.

115. White, M.T. and J. Gamm, *Informed consent for research on stored blood and tissue samples: a survey of institutional review board practices.* Account Res, 2002. 9(1): p. 1-16.

116. Austin, M.A., S.E. Harding, and C.E. McElroy, *Monitoring ethical, legal, and social issues in developing population genetic databases.* Genet Med, 2003. 5(6): p. 451-7.

117. Weil, C., et al., *OHRP compliance oversight letters: an update.* IRB, 2010. 32(2): p. 1-6.

118. Taylor, P.L., *State payer mandates to cover care in US oncology trials: do science and ethics matter?* J Natl Cancer Inst, 2010. 102(6): p. 376-90.

119. Sirotin, N., et al., *IRBs and ethically challenging protocols: views of IRB chairs about useful resources.* IRB, 2010. 32(5): p. 10-9.

120. Sacca, L., *The uncontrolled clinical trial: scientific, ethical, and practical reasons for being.* Intern Emerg Med, 2010. 5(3): p. 201-4.

121. Barrett, R., *Strategies for promoting the scientific integrity of nursing research in clinical settings.* J Nurses Staff Dev, 2010. 26(5): p. 200-5; quiz 260-7.

122. Kodish, E., et al., *Ethical issues in phase I oncology research: a comparison of investigators and institutional review board chairpersons.* J Clin Oncol, 1992. 10(11): p. 1810-6.

123. Paasche-Orlow, M.K. and F.L. Brancati, *Assessment of medical school institutional review board policies regarding compensation of subjects for research-related injury.* Am J Med, 2005. 118(2): p. 175-80.

124. Stevens, T., et al., *Palliative care research protocols: a special case for ethical review?* Palliat Med, 2003. 17(6): p. 482-90.

125. Campbell, E.G., et al., *Characteristics of medical school faculty members serving on institutional review boards: results of a national survey.* Acad Med, 2003. 78(8): p. 831-6.

126. Wolf, L.E., M. Croughan, and B. Lo, *The challenges of IRB review and human subjects protections in practice-based research.* Med Care, 2002. 40(6): p. 521-9.

127. Wolf, L.E., J.F. Walden, and B. Lo, *Human subjects issues and IRB review in practice-based research.* Ann Fam Med, 2005. 3 Suppl 1: p. S30-7.

128. Coleman, C.H. and M.C. Bouesseau, *How do we know that research ethics committees are really working? The neglected role of outcomes assessment in research ethics review.* BMC Med Ethics, 2008. 9: p. 6.

129. Schuppli, C.A. and D. Fraser, *Factors influencing the effectiveness of research ethics committees.* J Med Ethics, 2007. 33(5): p. 294-301.

130. Wichman, A., et al., *Protecting human subjects in the NIH's Intramural Research Program: a draft instrument to evaluate convened meetings of its IRBs.* IRB, 2006. 28(3): p. 7-10.

131. Angell, E.L., et al., *An analysis of decision letters by research ethics committees: the ethics/scientific quality boundary examined.* Qual Saf Health Care, 2008. 17(2): p. 131-6.

132. Dixon-Woods, M., et al., *Written work: the social functions of Research Ethics Committee letters.* Soc Sci Med, 2007. 65(4): p. 792-802.

133. MacNeil, S.D. and C.V. Fernandez, *Attitudes of research ethics board chairs towards disclosure of research results to participants: results of a national survey.* J Med Ethics, 2007. 33(9): p. 549-53.

134. Macneil, S.D. and C.V. Fernandez, *Informing research participants of research results: analysis of Canadian university based research ethics board policies.* J Med Ethics, 2006. 32(1): p. 49-54.

135. Vandenbrouke, J.P., *More on the LIFE study.* Lancet, 2003. 261: p. 532-3.

136. van der Meer, J.W., et al., *Independent medical research.* Neth J Med, 2007. 65(4): p. 124-6.

137. Kjaerdgard, L.L. and B. Als-Nielson, *Association between competing interests and authors' conclusions: epidemiological study of randomised clinical trials published in the BMJ.* BMJ, 2002. 325: p. 24.

138. Lexchin, J., et al., *Pharmaceutical industry sponsorship and research outcome and quality: systematic review.* BMJ, 2003. 326: p. 1167-70.

139. Ridker, P.M. and J. Torres, *Reported outcomes in major cardivascular clinical trials funded by for-profit and not-for-profit organizations.* JAMA, 2006. 295: p. 2270-4.

140. Vandenbrouke, J.P., *Was the LIFE trial independent?* Lancet, 2002. 360: p. 1171.

141. Choudry, N.K., H.T. Stelfox, and A.S. Detsky, *Relationships between authors of clinical practice guidelines and the pharmaceutical industry.* JAMA, 2002. 287: p. 612-7.

142. Hall, M.A., *The theory and practice of disclosing HMO physician incentives.* Law Contemp Probl, 2002. 64: p. 207-40.

APPENDIX A. EVIDENCE TABLES

Author/ Year	Study Design	Participants	Findings
Lo, 2000[100]	Analysis of COI policies	10 US Medical Schools receiving the largest amount of research funding from the NIH: Baylor, Columbia, Harvard, Johns Hopkins, UCLA, UCSF, U. of Penn, U. of Washington, Washington U., Yale	- all policies required disclosure of financial interests, including stock and stock options and income from salary, honorariums and consulting fees. -5 required disclosure of all financial interest, regardless of the value -5 required disclosure if > $10,000 -Further info on person required to disclose, to whom to disclose, prohibited interests
McCrary, 2000[99]	Deductive content analysis on COI policies to evaluate the documents according to certain domains	All US Medical Schools (n=127), and other research institutions (n=170) that received more than $5 million in total grants annually from the NIH or NHS, 48 journals in basic science and clinical medicine, and 17 federal agencies N= 250 institutions, 47 journals, 16 federal agencies	-250 institutions: 6% had no COI policies 91% adhered to the federal threshold for disclosure, 9% exceeded federal guidelines -Journals: 43% had policies requiring disclosure of COI -Federal agencies: 25% had policies that explicitly addressed COI 15/16- relied primarily on institutional discretion -Further info on 235 institutions with disclosure requirements including: type of conflict, person (or entity) with interest requiring initial disclosure, party to which initial disclosure must be made, when disclosure is required, how disclosure should be managed, penalty for nondisclosure.
Weinfurt, 2010[13]	Survey of financial conflict policies	199 sites in US with at least partial commercial sponsorship that contributed participants to phase 3 clinical trials, the results of which were published in either JAMA or NEJM. Response rate/(n) = 66% (61) for academic medical centers, 37% (77) for non-academic medical centers, and 27% (61) for nonacademic outpatient settings	Compared academic medical centers/ nonacademic medical centers/ outpatient nonacademic sites in various domains, including: Follow formal written policy on investigator financial relationships- 97%/ 87%/ 44% Also, whether required to report financial relationships, type of IRB review, the persons or groups with role in review of investigators' financial relationships, whether consideration of reasonableness of per capita payment amounts, whether institution has nonemployee investigators and reviews financial relationships of nonemployee investigators, whether institution uses monetary threshold below which there is no review of investigators/ financial relationships, whether institution uses NIH threshold, and whether there are prohibited financial relationships.
Weinfurt, 2007[96]	Focus groups, cognitive interviews and expert panel development and revision	16 focus groups with healthy adults, adults with mild chronic/ serious illness, parents of healthy/ seriously ill children; cognitive interviews (n=10) with a convenience sample from primary care clinic; an expert panel discussion	-developed model disclosure statement. included generic disclosure statement (person leading study might benefit financially), specific disclosure statement (how might benefit financially- including descriptions of salary support, money received outside of the study, per capita payments, finders' fees restricted to research uses, unrestricted finders' fees, researcher or university holding a patent or equity

Author/Year	Study Design	Participants	Findings
Weinfurt, 2006[92]	Descriptive assessment of COI policies, most collected via publicly available information on internet	123 academic medical centers, with IRBs. Response rate/ (n) = 98% (120)	-goals of disclosure of COI should include: promoting autonomy, avoid legal liability, and deterrence. -majority of policies most consistent with goal of avoiding legal liability. -48% mentioned disclosure to potential research subjects. Of these, 58% required or suggested verbatim language for the informed consent document. -all required disclosure of the study sponsor, 38% required nature of financial relationship disclosed. -18% specified disclosing how funds allocated. -4% required notification that protocol reviewed by COIC or other administrative body. -5% made reference to nonfinancial interests.
Weinfurt, 2006[97]	Scripted interviews	10 US academic medical centers, 10 independent hospitals, 10 unaffiliated research entities N= 23 IRB chairs, 14 COIC chairs and 8 investigators	Coding of interview transcripts led to comparisons between investigators, IRB chairs and COIC chairs regarding circumstances in which conflicts of interest should be disclosed, rationale for or benefits of disclosure, information to be disclosed, negative effects or barriers to disclosure, timing of disclosure.
Campbell, 2006[93]	Survey on financial relationships between IRB members and industry	Random sample of 893 IRB members at 100 academic institutions in US. Response Rate/ (n), 67.2% (574)	78 reported at least one protocol came before their IRB with which they had COI 58% always disclosed the relationship to an IRB official 8% sometimes did 12% rarely did 23% never did Of the 62 who were voting members 65% never voted on a protocol 5% rarely did 11% sometimes did 19% always did
Vogeli, 2009[95]	Anonymous survey of IRB chairs	IRB chairs at the most research-intensive medical institutions in US Response Rate/(n) = 71.7% (211)	68% have written policy defining COI 22% did not 9% did not know Further info on to whom to report, how disclosure managed, confidence in policies/ procedures, how conflicts managed

Maintaining Research Integrity: A Systematic Review of the Role of the IRB in Managing Conflict of Interest

Author/Year	Study Design	Participants	Findings
Wolf, 2007[91]	Assessment of IRB policies regarding COI, most collected from IRB websites and IRB representatives	121 medical schools receiving NIH funding in fiscal year 2003	74% had written policies 79% of those defined what constituted a COI 10 required any financial interest disclosed 23 only > $10,000 4 significant (undefined) financial interests 14 no definition of a financial interest 99% referred to all IRB members, 1% only IRB chairs, 14% IRB staff, 20% ad hoc reviewers and consultants, 4% guests 4/92 address failure to comply
Brody, 2003[98]	Self-report questionnaire with 12 questions relating to policy for disclosure, institutional management of disclosed possible COIs, action by institution when COI is not disclosed	158 senior investigators, 297 senior research administrators, 195 bioethicists, 17 journal editors and 7 agency administrators	Overall, all supported disclosure to IRBs, research subjects, journals and funding agencies Only the bioethicists were strongly supportive of including research subjects
Weinfurt, 2009[94]	Examined 5 years of empirical data from the Conflict of Interest Notification study, to formulate 6 suggested goals of disclosure	n/a, data from study	6 goals of disclosure: promoting informed decision making, respecting participants' perceived right to know, establishing or maintaining trust, minimizing risk of legal liability, deterring troubling financial relationships, protecting research participants' welfare

APPENDIX B. PEER REVIEW COMMENTS TABLE

	Reviewer	Comment	Response
Are the objectives, scope, and methods for this review clearly described?	1	None	No response needed
	2	None	No response needed
	3	Yes – though the method of pursuing the item with multiple publications and no VA policy might be an odd way to set priorities.	No response needed
	4	Clearly described, but I believe fatally flawed in their limited scope.	See below for specific comments to specific critiques
	5	None	No response needed
	6	Overall, the purpose of the review are clearly defined with good documentation on the methods, search terms, inclusion/exclusion criteria, etc.	No response needed
	7	None	No response needed
Is there any indication of bias in our synthesis of the evidence?	1	None	No response needed
	2	None	No response needed
	3	None	No response needed
	4	As indicated in my response to question 4. below, I believe that the authors have been even-handed in how they have synthesized what evidence they have collected.	No response needed
		I believe there are a number of important biases that resulted from how they have cast their review net that should really be addressed.	See below
		I suspect that Key question #1 is incomplete, and had they incorporated additional literatures as I have suggested below, that where they might have gone with Key question #2 might be entirely different than it is currently.	See below
	5	None	No response needed
	6	No indication of bias.	No response needed
	7	No bias was introduced from the methods but given the change in implementation of COI policies in the last decade, a more refined analysis should be considered. For example, dividing the time period into first five years versus second five years might be illuminating.	Unfortunately, we were not able to operationalize this good suggestion, since only one of the studies published during the second five year time frame collected data during the prior five years. All the other more recently published studies had data from before 2005.

	Reviewer	Comment	Response
Are there any published or unpublished studies that we may have overlooked?	1	I don't know of any "studies" that were missed, however, I think there are probably relevant white papers and other commentaries on these subjects that would have been relevant (e.g., from AAMC, PRIM&R, and AAHRPP, NIH and other Federal entities).	We searched the websites of each of these organizations and identified only COI policies or position papers, no empiric studies of COI. We added text to the methods regarding this.
	2	Pape T, Jaffe NO, Savage T, Collins E, Warden D Unresolved legal and ethical issues in research of adults with severe traumatic brain injury: Analysis of an ongoing protocol. J Rehabil Res & Devel. 2004;41(2):155-74.	We reviewed this paper and it describes legal and ethical issues with respect to adults with traumatic brain injury. It does not deal with COI and therefore we did not include it in our review.
	3	At least, I don't know of any and the methods seem comprehensive.	No response needed
	4	I've indicated a number of studies that I think may have been overlooked – but I have not tried to be exhaustive about this.	No response needed
	5	None	No response needed
	6	None	No response needed
	7	I believe there is literature expressing the opinion that disclosing financial COIs in the consent document or process might have undue influence if participants think the study is better designed or safer because the investigator has an interest.	We didn't find such studies and without a specific citation we can't check on this.

Maintaining Research Integrity: A Systematic Review of the Role of the IRB in Managing Conflict of Interest

	Reviewer	Comment	Response
Please write additional suggestions or comments below. If applicable, please indicate the page and line numbers from the draft report.	1	Policy development on VHA research conflict of interest has been underway for quite some time. I am surprised the authors do not seem to be aware of that fact. Dr. Brenda Cuccherini is the contact person in ORD. Also, the authors should look at the conflict of interest issues covered in VHA Handbook 1200.05.	The relevant sections of VHA Handbook 1200.05 are as follows: Disclosing Conflicts of Interests. This means disclosing to the IRB any potential, actual, or perceived conflict of interest of a financial, professional, or personal nature that may affect any aspect of the research, and complying with all applicable VA and other Federal requirements regarding conflict of interest. (p20) Conflict of Interest. No IRB may have a member participate in the IRB's initial or continuing review of any study in which the member has a conflicting interest, except to provide information requested by IRB (38 CFR 16.107(e)). (p38) Conflict of Interest. The IRB must ensure that steps to manage, reduce, or eliminate potential, actual, or perceived conflicts of interest related to all aspects of the research (financial, role (investigator-patient relationships), and other professional, institutional, or personal roles) have been taken. (p46) While these directions articulate general goals, it is the specifics of how they are operationalized that is the question of interest.
	2	COI as it relates to investigators seems to be monitored carefully now. Investigators are asked to disclose potential and actual COIs. The question of COI amongst IRB members and reviewers is not discussed as much. I think the authors have hit on a relative weakness in the system and further exploration is needed in this area.	No response needed
	3	If I were asked to consider the sources of conflict of interest in research review, the first thing that would come to mind did not even arise in this review. I would have first thought of the conflict of interest in the IRB with having to consider and defend the institutional interests of the sponsoring institution, as well as the well-being and autonomy of research subjects. This is a pervasive conflict of interest and may well be undercutting the IRB endeavor – since many IRBs seem to act more to defend their home institution from harm than to defend research subjects. I am sure I have read others commenting on this, though I don't know exactly where to point to without some additional research in the literature. Is it really the case that this did not arise in the literature search? Or is it that this did come up but was ruled out of scope for this project?	We did not find empiric studies of this. It may exist in policy statements but reviewing policy statements was not our scope.

Reviewer	Comment	Response
Please write additional suggestions or comments below. If applicable, please indicate the page and line numbers from the draft report.	4	The author's decision to focus on conflict of interest issues in research seems to have been driven largely by the number of articles they uncovered specifically in the PubMed database on the various potential issues of interest identified under the heading of **Key Question #1**. This is a potentially problematic decision for the entire review since the only literature database searched here was PubMed. This makes the review far from systematic. In particular, the PubMed database would miss a great deal of the social science literature on these topics. Inclusion of the main social science, legal, educational and perhaps humanities databases (e.g. Psychology Abstracts, Sociological Abstracts, Lexis, Westlaw, ERIC, etc.) would likely have uncovered additional literature on these specific topics as well as identifying additional topics that may have provided alternative foci of interest for this review. As one example, my sense is that there has been a great deal of discussion within humanities literature about what defines and distinguishes research activities from quality improvement activities. As another example, there's been voluminous discussion within a variety of social science literature's about whether IRB's that are predominantly biomedical in their composition and dispositions provide adequate and appropriate review of social science studies. This would seem to be a particularly relevant issue for the VA HSR&D program, since much of the research in that program employs social science methods and perspectives. The reviewers rejected a focus on the distinctions between research and quality improvement initiatives as a topic of interest for their in-depth review addressing Key question #2. They justify this decision by pointing out that VA has recently offered definitions of these concepts, which they include on pages 9 and 10 of the report. To this reviewer, the VA definitions seem to offer an equivocal position on the distinction between research and quality improvement initiatives, and do not seem to offer clear guidance to researchers or IRBs about the conditions under which various systematic activities should be exempted from IRB review. I say this as both a researcher, and as someone with a decade's worth of IRB service under my belt. It strikes me that this VA "policy" could in fact use some improvements, which might begin with a review of two very recent publications on this topic: 1) Emanuel and Menikoff in NEJM[1]; 2) Selker et al. – Discussion Paper of a working group drawn from the "Clinical Effectiveness Research Innovation Collaborative of the IOM Roundtable on Value & Science-Driven Healthcare."[2] On page v, the authors describe one of the topics uncovered in their literature search as "payment to patients." Here again is an issue that likely would have been more voluminously represented in the literature had social science databases been included in the author's search. I suspect that a search of those databases would have uncovered a great deal of discussion regarding not just payments to patients but more broadly speaking numerous issues around use of "incentives for research/study subjects." In survey-based research, the study of subject incentives if practically a cottage industry, and at least some of that work has taken up concerns with the ethics questions involved. The list of articles classified by the authors under the "miscellaneous" heading is surprisingly brief. Again I think this is likely indicative of the unfortunate decision to restrict their literature review to the PubMed database.	While we respect this reviewer's input, the decisions about where to focus the detailed review was made in consultation with VA Central Office stakeholders and is not something we can change. We reviewed the New Republic article by Lessig and were not as convinced as this reviewer that this is on target for this topic. The example used of JAMA's COI policy and the effect it had on a JAMA critic doesn't seem particularly relevant to investigators or IRBs dealing with possible financial interest in the research studies they conduct or review. If the point is that transparency of COI policies can have unintended consequences, that we agree with, but it is for empiric research to determine whether and to what magnitude such unintended consequences occur. We did devote a section of the review to potential harms of disclosure. We searched the internet for information on the VCU case and there has been no peer-reviewed publication about it, only one letter or commentary in BMJ.

Reviewer	Comment	Response
4 (Cont'd)	Though it may have to do with search terms they have selected as well. As but one example of something I had expected to see here but did not is some very nice empirical work by Keith-Spiegel and colleagues on the issues of relationships between researchers and IRB's that is directly relevant to issues of research integrity.3,4 **Issues within the portion of the review dealing specifically with conflicts of interest.** The reviewed literature on COI seems to have focused almost exclusively on the issue of disclosure thereof. A very fundamental problem with this is that it jumps directly over the more obvious, but obviously more fraught approaches to COI emphasized by the two prominent reports (of the IOM and NIH) referenced on p. 2 of the current report. Specifically, both of those statements place emphasis primarily on the elimination and avoidance of conflicts of interest, and the active management of such conflicts where they cannot be eliminated or avoided, perhaps through formal means such as the creation of COI committees. Only lastly do they mention disclosure as an ameliorative, suggesting that they do not see this as a sufficient approach in and of itself. It would be striking had this just been an oversight of the report authors, but it is an astonishing blind-spot in the literature if there has been no empirical research into this. That the avoidance of COI has not been, and is not the focus of thought and discussion on this topic suggests that the community has yet to come truly to grips with the need to engage the problem at its roots. This reviewer is increasingly convinced that disclosure itself may be a really bad idea and likely has unanticipated consequences in undermining public trust, not preserving it. My own thinking on this topic has been influence by a 2009 article on the topic, written by Lawrence Lessig and published in The New Republic.5 Lessig makes what I find a very compelling case against relying on "transparency" as an antiseptic with respect to misbehaviors of those in government, arguing that such transparency would very likely undermine public trust and not accomplish its primary objective. I think his points translate largely into the realm of research and public trust as well. I was also very struck to see that the discussion of conflict of interest seemed to focus nearly exclusively on the issue of financial conflicts of interest that are introduced by individual researcher or IRB member involvement with industry in particular. Has there truly been no examination of institutional conflicts of interest (such as between University leadership decisions and funders, whether private OR public) as they may adversely impact the integrity of research? As one example, did the Martinson et al. 2009 article in Academic Medicine6 not get captured in the initial net that was cast? Has there been nothing published in the academic literature about the startling institutional conflicts of interest that were unearthed in 2008 between Philip-Morris and Virginia Commonwealth University? That controversy initially embroiled Frank Macrina (who was VP at VCU at the time), himself the author of the most widely cited textbook on responsible conduct of research!
Was there no empirical work on the potentially conflicted nature of IRB service itself? Aside from the requisite community members and perhaps professional ethicists, most members of "local" IRB's are drawn from their own employing institution. This can readily put them in a conflicted position between loyalty to their employer and loyalty to the study subjects involved in the studies they are reviewing. I have witnessed this conflict first hand on a number of occasions in my own IRB service. One might view this as a concern about institutional conflicts of interest, which is again, another topic that I had expected to see arise in this review which is entirely absent.	

Maintaining Research Integrity: A Systematic Review of the Role of the IRB in Managing Conflict of Interest

Evidence-based Synthesis Program

	Reviewer	Comment	Response
Please write additional suggestions or comments below. If applicable, please indicate the page and line numbers from the draft report.	4 (Cont'd)	http://vabio.blogspot.com/2008/05/nyt-tobacco-research-is-secret-at-vcu.html	
		http://www2.richmond.com/business/2008/oct/01/vcu-report-on-tobacco-research-due-today-ar-627812/?referer=http://www.google.com/search&shorturl=http://bit.ly/dGHzhh	
		Minor points:	
		What is the correct number of articles identified under the topic of when quality improvement initiatives are considered research? At the top of page v the report indicates 31 whereas in the middle of page 10 indicates 32.	
		References:	We obtained and reviewed the references cited by the reviewer. References 1,2,3 and 5 are opinions or commentaries and do not contain data and are therefore not included in our review. Reference 4 describes the result of a survey to identify the attributes of an "ideal" IRB from the perspective of researchers. While the results are interesting (the most highly valued item was "an IRB that reviews protocols in a timely fashion") they do not deal directly with the issue of COI or how it is applied. Reference 6 is a survey of 5000 randomly selected faculty from which 1703 yielded usable data, and while the results are revealing in terms of the relationship between funding source and potentially inappropriate behaviors, it does not deal with conflict of interest policies per se or their application.
		1. Emanuel EJ, Menikoff J. Reforming the Regulations Governing Research with Human Subjects. *N Engl J Med*. 2011. Available at: http://www.ncbi.nlm.nih.gov/entrez/query.fcgi?cmd=Retrieve&db=PubMed&dopt=Citation&list_uids=21787202.
2. Selker HP, Grossman C, Adams A, et al. The Common Rule and Continuous Improvement in Health Care: A Learning Health System Perspective - Institute of Medicine. Available at: http://iom.edu/Global/Perspectives/2012/CommonRule.aspx. Accessed February 8, 2012.
3. Keith-Spiegel P, Koocher GP. The IRB Paradox: Could the Protectors Also Encourage Deceit? *Ethics & Behavior*. 2005;15:339–349.
4. Keith-Spiegel P, Koocher GP, Tabachnick B. What Scientists Want from Their Research Ethics Committee. *Journal of Empirical Research on Human Research Ethics*. 2006;1:67–82.
5. Lessig L. Against Transparency: The perils of openness in government. *The New Republic*. 2009;(October 9). Available at: http://www.tnr.com/article/books-and-arts/against-transparency. Accessed March 4, 2012.
6. Martinson BC, Crain AL, Anderson MS, De Vries R. Institutions' Expectations for Researchers' Self-Funding, Federal Grant Holding and Private Industry Involvement: Manifold Drivers of Self-Interest and Researcher Behavior. *Academic Medicine*. 2009;84:1491–1499.	
	5	This draft report by Shekelle et al., detailed the results of their reviews of the literature from January 1, 2000, to February 11, 201, on issues related to the Institutional Review Board (IRB) including quality improvement initiatives, conflict of interest (COI) in research, multisite studies requiring multiple IRB approvals, and genetic research. A total of 116 articles were identified and reviewed. Although more articles were related to issues related to multisite studies requiring multiple IRB reviews (41 articles) and quality improvement projects (31 articles), the authors focused on issues related to research COI and IRB (11 articles), as currently VHA does not have a research COI policy. The review and analysis of the literature appeared to be adequate, and the draft report appeared to be well written. There are, however, a number of concerns: 1. As pointed out by the authors, the number of articles reviewed for the main topic, i.e., research COI and IRB, was small (i.e., 11 articles). In addition, there were substantial limitations in some of these articles including small sample sizes and low survey response rates. As a result, the draft report does not provide sufficient information/evidence to guide VHA policy makers in developing a research COI policy.	1. This is correct. The purpose of the review was not to assist VA in developing COI policies per se, but rather to examine the potential challenges in their application.

Maintaining Research Integrity: A Systematic Review of the Role of the IRB in Managing Conflict of Interest

Evidence-based Synthesis Program

Reviewer	Comment	Response
5 (Contd)	2. The authors repeatedly used the term "multisite institutional research board challenge." (see pages iv and 7) First of all, I believe they meant "multisite institutional review board (IRB) challenge." In addition, I believe they were talking about the challenge presented by multisite studies that required multiple IRB review and approval. The term multisite IRB is used for an IRB that covers a number of research facilities such as VA Central IRB. For example, VISN 4 has a VISN4 Multisite IRB located at the Coatesville VAMC that is being used as the IRB of record for not only Coatesville VAMC, but also for Wilkes-Barre VAMC (and Lebanon VAMC, and Erie VAMC in the past).	2. This sentence has been rephrased.
	3. On Page 9, the authors attempted to summarize VHA Handbook 1058.05 in Table 2. However, it really missed the essence of the Handbook. The following provides a better summary of the VHA Handbook 1058.05 entitled, "VHA Operations Activities that May Constitute Research." Health care operations activities such as quality assurance and quality improvement projects differ from research in that health care operations activities are specifically designed to support the operations of a health care institution, while research is specifically designed to contribute to generalizable knowledge (i.e., to expand the knowledge base of a scientific discipline or other scholarly field of study). Both health care operations activity and research utilize systematic investigation to achieve their objectives. Similar to research, the results of health care operations activity may be published in scientific journals and ultimately expand scientific knowledge base. Thus, neither systematic investigation nor publication effectively distinguishes health care operations activity from research. However, when a health care operations activity goes beyond its purpose of supporting the operations of a health care institution by adding elements specifically designed to expand the knowledge base of a scientific discipline or other scholarly field of study, the activity constitutes research.	3. This text was added
	4. On Page v, 3rd paragraph, it was stated that "Across studies, the amount of payment appeared related to the magnitude of the procedures to be performed or the time to participate in the study." However, on page 12, 1st paragraph, it was stated that "Across studies, there was, in general, no indication that the payment was related to the procedures to be performed or the time commitment required to participate in the study." (see also Pages vii and 23) Which one is correct?	4. This was a typographical error, it is "unrelated"
	5. On Page 2, 1st paragraph, it was stated that "IRBs also distinguish what constitutes a research study with human participation (i.e., an intervention that potentially subjects a patient to risk without guarantee of likely benefit and therefore requires IRB review) from quality improvement initiatives that do not directly involve participants." This statement is misleading. Human research does not have to directly involve participants. Likewise, quality improvement initiatives may directly involve human participants.	5. These revisions have been made.
	6. The numbers on page 6 do not add up! The number of references excluded should be 47, instead of 44 as stated in Pages iv and 6. In addition, it should be pointed out that the same two articles were included in Conflicts of Interest (N=11) as well as Genetics (N=8).	6. This sentence has been rephrased

	Reviewer	Comment	Response
Please write additional suggestions or comments below. If applicable, please indicate the page and line numbers from the draft report.	5 (Cont'd)	7. The second paragraph on Page 19 should have a new subtitle, as it does not belong to either "Who has Policies on Disclosure?" or "Conflict of Interest within an IRB." I suggest a subtitle such as "Which COI should be disclosed to Research participants?"	7. We have added to this section a modified version of this additional subtitle.
		8. Tables 1, 3, 4, 5 and 6 should be deleted, as they did not add any useful information. These references were already listed in Pages 28-35 under References.	8. We prefer to keep these in the text.
		9. On Page 15, there is a difference between "regulations" and "policies" or "guidelines." The NIH guidelines on financial conflict of interest are not "regulations."	9. According to NIH's website, the 2011 statements are "regulations" and so we continue to refer to them as such in the report. Please see: http://grants.nih.gov/grants/policy/coi/
		10. There were multiple typographical errors throughout the draft report (please see attached draft report in Track Change).	10. We identified and corrected the 3 typographical errors that were identified.
	6	Overall, this was a thorough summary of the literature. The use of frequencies in reporting articles and approaches helped convey the emphasis of the literature.	No response needed
	7	I put comments directly into the draft. The analysis and report are good. They should be published.	No response needed
Are there any clinical performance measures, programs, quality improvement measures, patient care services, or conferences that will be directly affected by this report? If so, please provide detail.	1	None since policy already is well on its way to being promulgated, and some of the areas identified in the document already are addressed in VHA Handbook 1200.05.	No response needed
	3	PRIMR, the current review of the Common Rule by OHRP	No response needed
	6	It is likely that the report will help clarify and remove obstacles in conducting research in clinical settings.	No response needed
	7	AAMC has a group called FOCI that meets several times annually. That would be a good conference. It could be presented at the annual AAHRPP conference and PRIM&R conferences.	No response needed
Please provide any recommendations on how this report can be revised to more directly address or assist implementation needs.	1	This document is not relevant since some of the studies cited are from several years ago, and VHA research conflict of interest policy based on current thinking in government, academia, and the private sector has already drafted.	We believe it remains a suitable topic for research to determine the degree of variability that may exist within VA in the application of COI policies by both researchers and IRBs.
	2	Additional information for IRB administrators might be in order. The authors may want to make a recommendation as to what types of COI should be monitored.	This is a good recommendation but is for Central Office policy makers and not within the scope of the evidence report.
	3	The literature searches might well be stand-alone reports in a journal like Hastings or Hastings IRB journal.	No response needed

Maintaining Research Integrity: A Systematic Review of the Role of the IRB in Managing Conflict of Interest

Evidence-based Synthesis Program

	Reviewer	Comment	Response
Please provide any recommendations on how this report can be revised to more directly address or assist implementation needs.	6	While the report did a good job of reviewing the literature, it would be helpful to have some mention or discussion about the implementation of the policies and the extent that how something is implemented (e.g., a conflicts of interest policy) may ultimately impact the overall effectiveness of a policy. The general emphasis—which was appropriate given the question—was on what the policies were, but the report leaves the reader with the impression that IRB and COI issues, for example, are primarily about defining the policy.	This important point was added to the future research.
Please provide us with contact details of any additional individuals/ stakeholders who should be made aware of this report.	1	Dr. Brenda Cuccherini, ORD	No response needed
	5	Dr, Brenda Cuccherini, Office of Research and Development	No response needed
	7	Ann Bonham, AAMC abonham@aamc.org I assume you have contacts at NIH.	No response needed

Additional Comments

Reviewer	Comment	Response
8	I agree with reviewer 9's main point as well. Since this is synthesizing evidence it would be appropriate to include some reference to the aggregated findings in the section below adding a very brief review (if possible at this late hour). Just an acknowledgement of the problem in a brief few lines should do it. Multisite Institutional Research Board Challenges We identified 41 articles that dealt with the challenges of having to submit a research protocol to IRBs at multiple institutions. Most were descriptive studies of how the same application was reviewed by different IRBs. VA has recently implemented a process whereby multi-site VA studies can be reviewed by a single, centralized IRB. Consequently, a detailed review of this issue would not be helpful to VA. Thanks for all those working on this.	We have added a brief statement (page 8) on the general findings within this topic.
9	The report is quite useful. As a consequence of the ESP and another document that addresses COI that HSR&D recently received, I will pursue an evaluation of COI both at an IRB and research project peer review committee levels. A few comments are attached: The presentation is clear, relevant, and useful. My only comment relates to the framing of Q2: " … for which no current policy exits." This framing results in statements that, "a detailed review of this issue would not be helpful to VA." To me, this sentence doesn't make sense, since my response is quite the opposite, i.e., because VA has determined that the issues are important (i.e., specific policy was developed), a detailed evaluation of the literature is also very important. HOWEVER, I am NOT proposing that the ESP be revised. It is truly useful as is. Rather, I suggest that the Key Question, and the rationale for focusing on COI, be revised. A few text revisions here and there in the Exec Summary (and perhaps in the body of the report) should be sufficient. Bottom Line – Nicely done. I greatly appreciate the consistent, high quality of the ES reports.	The phrasing of this key question has been revised to better frame its intent.

www.ingramcontent.com/pod-product-compliance
Lightning Source LLC
Chambersburg PA
CBHW081617170526
45166CB00009B/3002